Infective Endocarditis

Edited by Peter Magnusson
and Robin Razmi

Published in London, United Kingdom

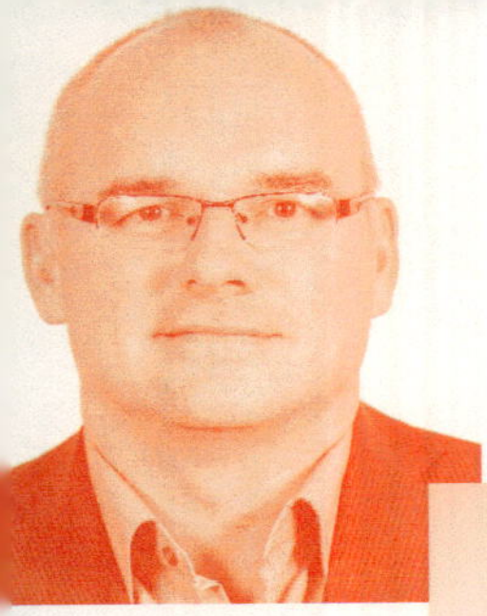
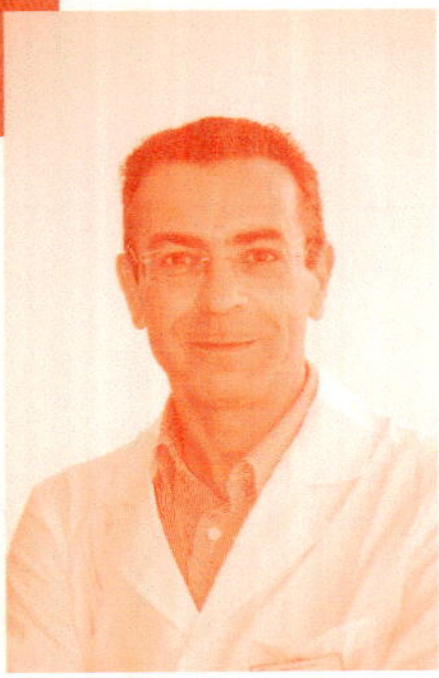
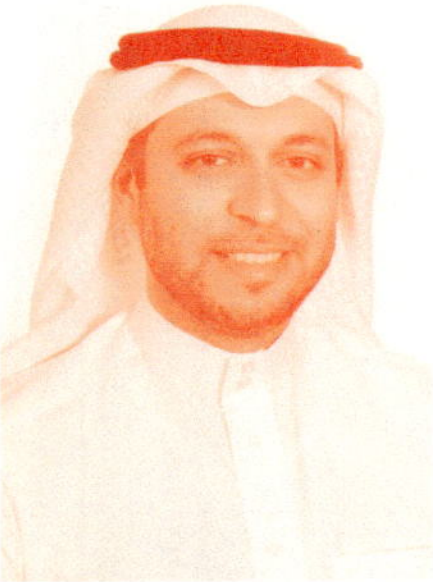
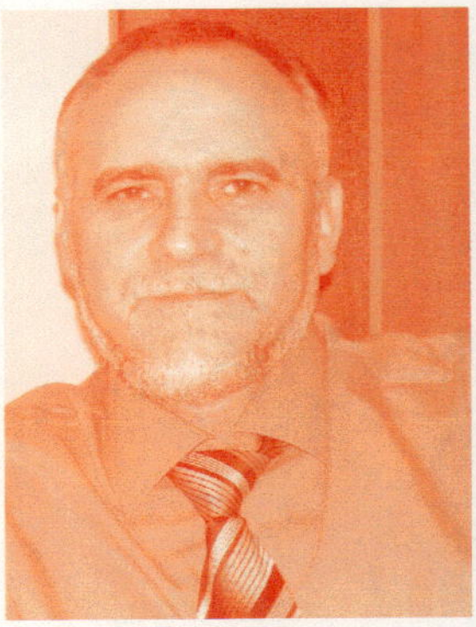
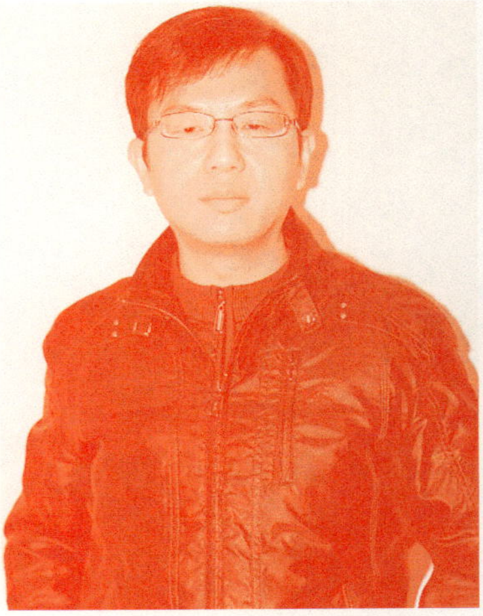
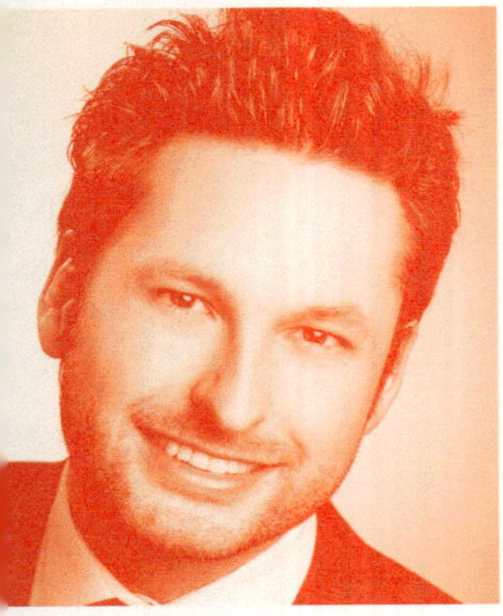
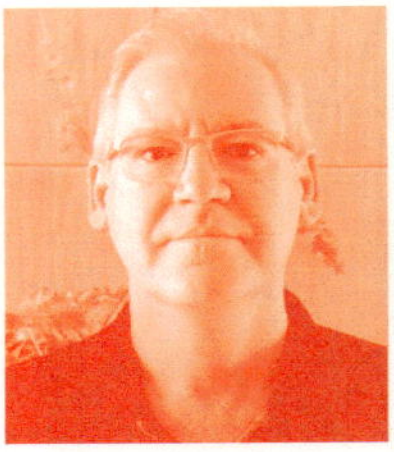

IntechOpen

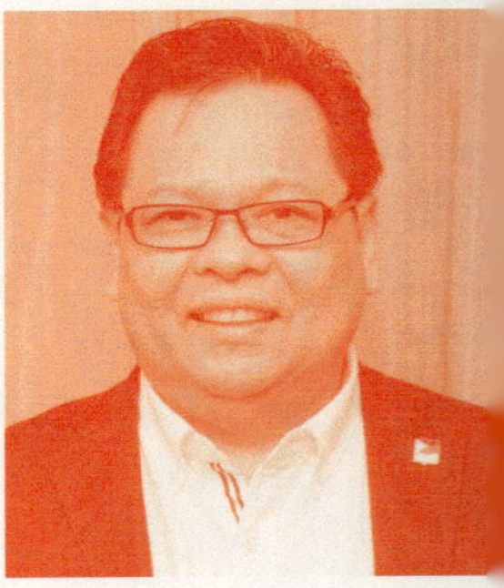
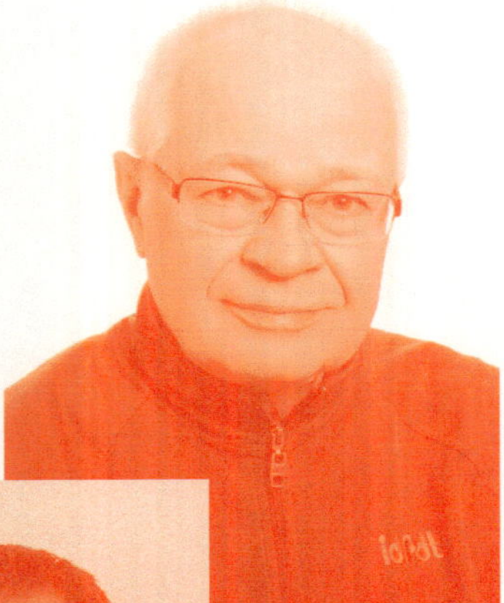
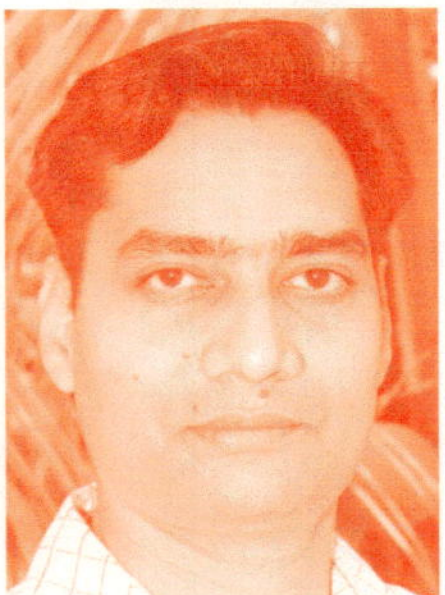
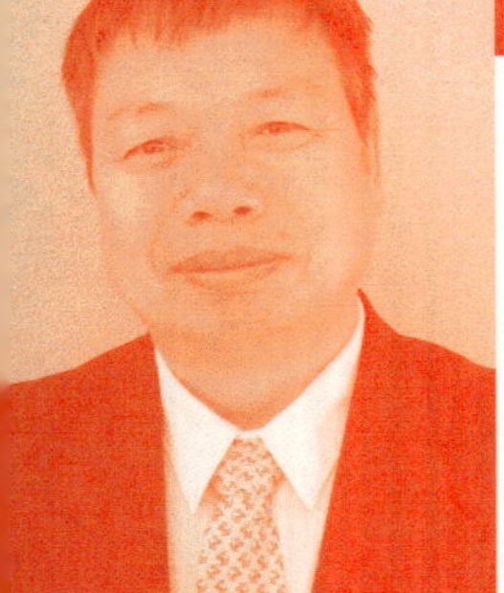
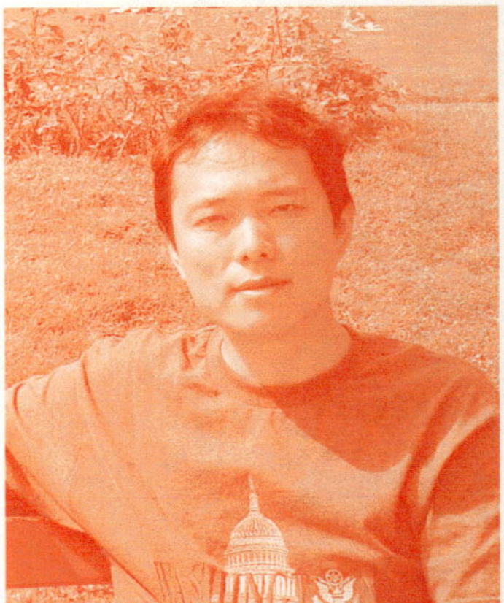
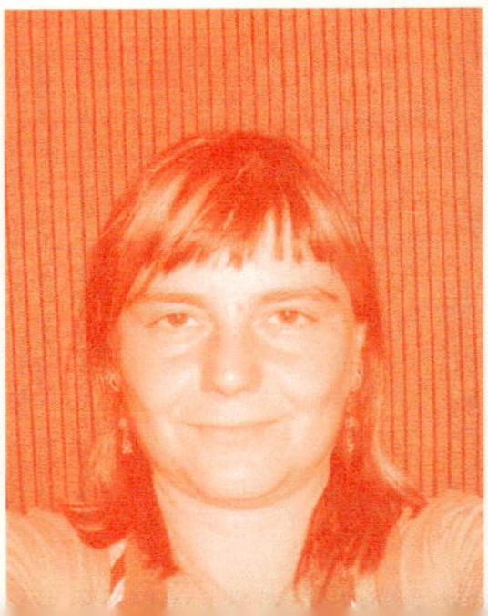

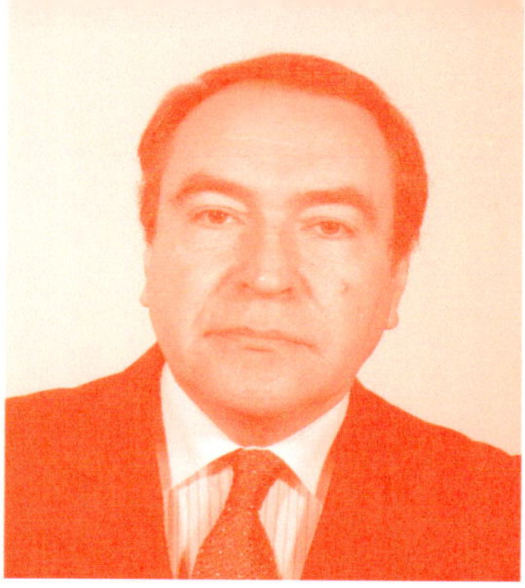

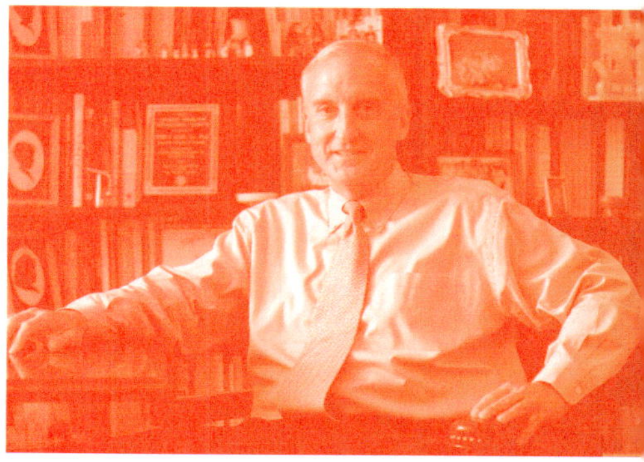

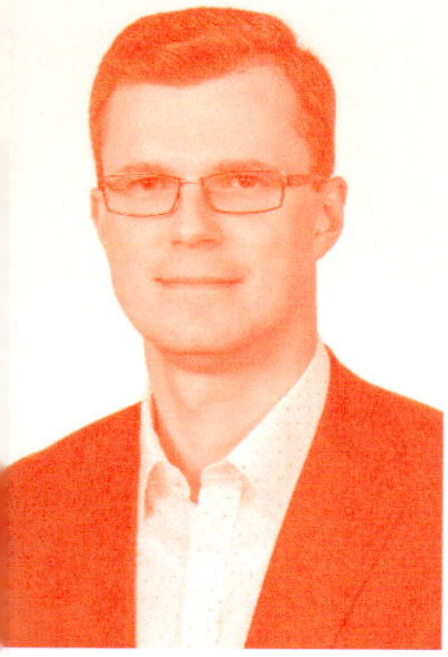

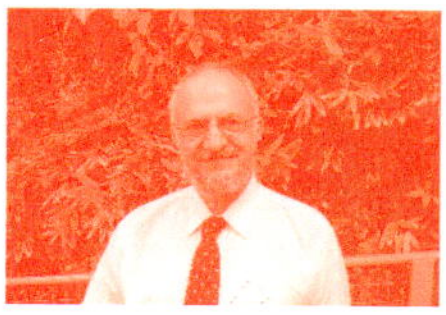

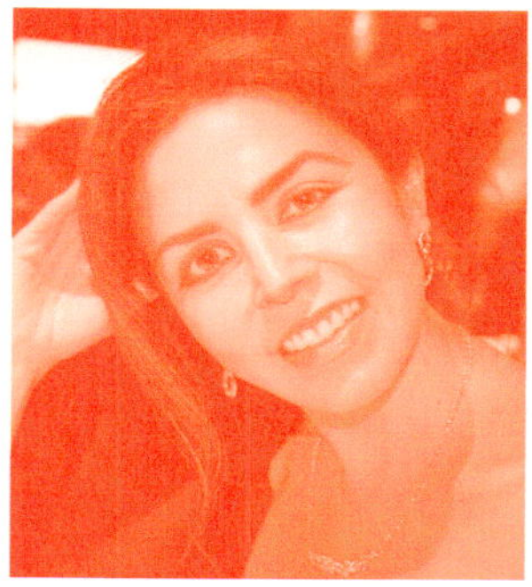

Supporting open minds since 2005

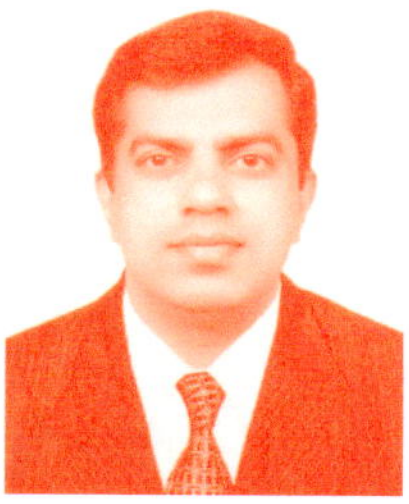

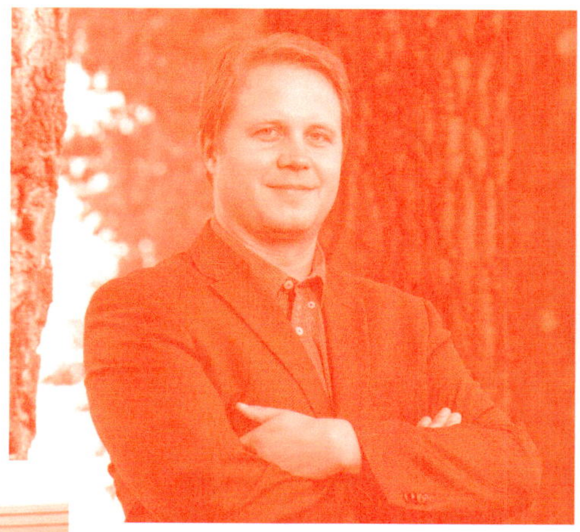

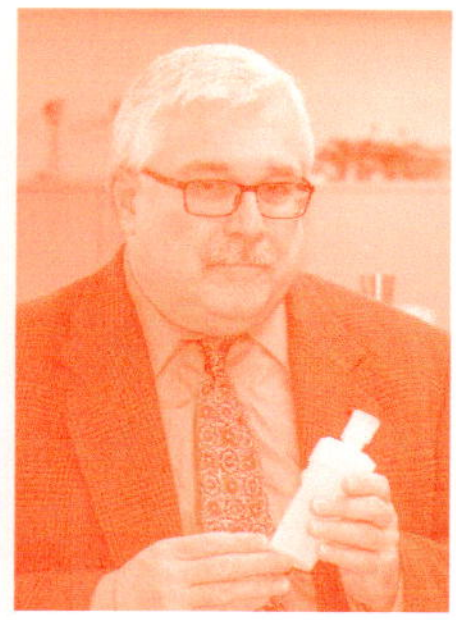

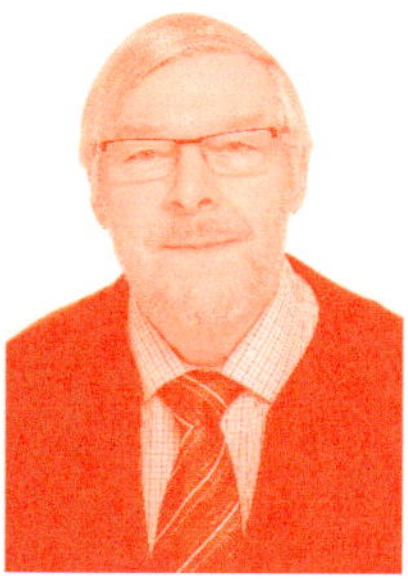

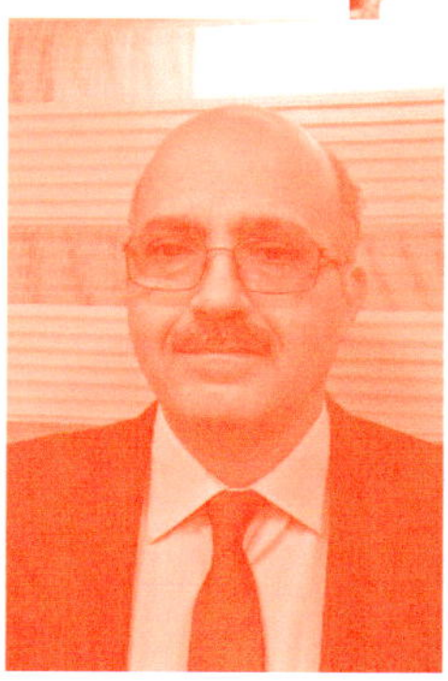

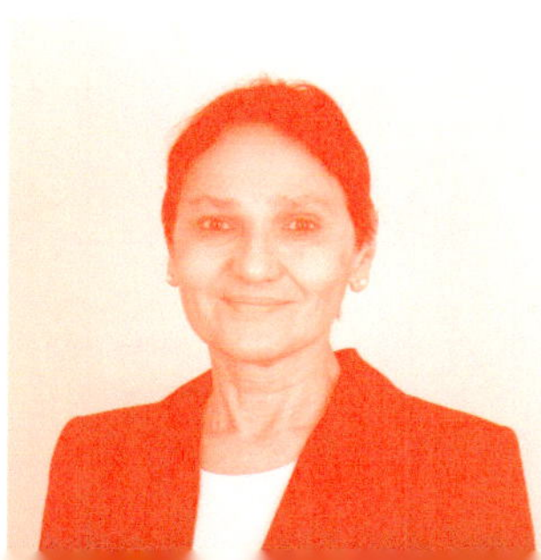

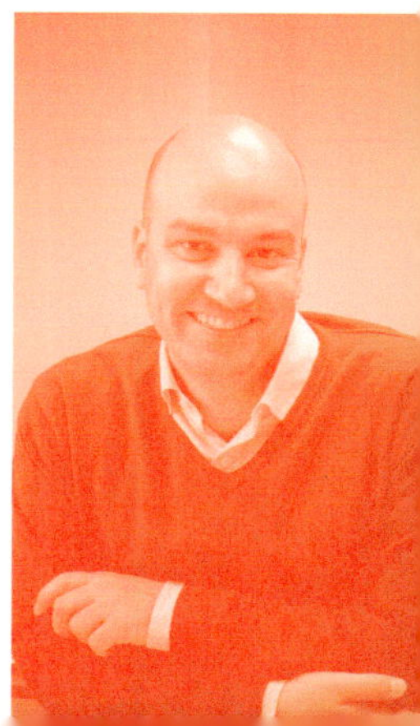

Infective Endocarditis
http://dx.doi.org/10.5772/intechopen.78176
Edited by Peter Magnusson and Robin Razmi

Contributors
Ruchika Meel, Pedro-Eduardo Alvarado-Rubio, Roberto Brugada, Cesar-Augusto Gonzalez-López, Alejandro Gonzalez, Pedro Eduardo Alvarado Avila, Angel Robles-Marhuenda, Carmen Busca-Arenzana, Luis Ramos-Ruperto, Jorge Alvarez-Troncoso, Gustav Mattsson, Måns Almqvist, Robin Razmi, Peter Michael Magnusson, Horatiu Moldovan, Adrian Fernando Narvaez Muñoz, Daniela Albina Ibarra Vargas

First published in London, United Kingdom, 2019 by IntechOpen
IntechOpen is the global imprint of INTECHOPEN LIMITED, registered in England and Wales, registration number: 11086078, The Shard, 25th floor, 32 London Bridge Street
London, SE19SG – United Kingdom
Printed in Croatia

British Library Cataloguing-in-Publication Data
A catalogue record for this book is available from the British Library

Additional hard and PDF copies can be obtained from orders@intechopen.com

Infective Endocarditis
Edited by Peter Magnusson and Robin Razmi
p. cm.
Print ISBN 978-1-78984-011-7
Online ISBN 978-1-78984-012-4
eBook (PDF) ISBN 978-1-78985-920-1

For EU product safety concerns:
IN TECH d.o.o., Prolaz Marije Krucifikse Kozulić 3, 51000 Rijeka, Croatia, info@intechopen.com or visit our website at intechopen.com.

Meet the editor

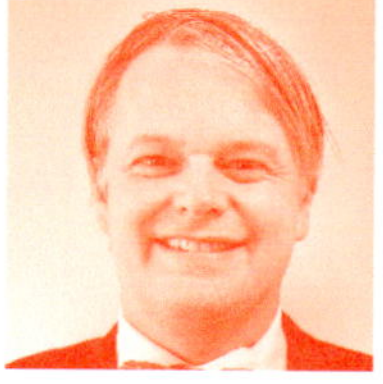

Peter Magnusson, MD, is a senior consultant in cardiology and active in research projects, including topics such as arrhythmia, cardiomyopathy, heart failure, and valvular disease. He is affiliated to the Karolinska Institute, Sweden, and the Center for Research and Development Region Gävleborg, Uppsala University, Sweden. Dr. Magnusson's research involves epidemiological studies, qualitative methods, observational studies, and randomized controlled trials. He is passionate about teaching and supervision, especially in academic projects. Currently, he is striving for implementation of research findings in the health care system.

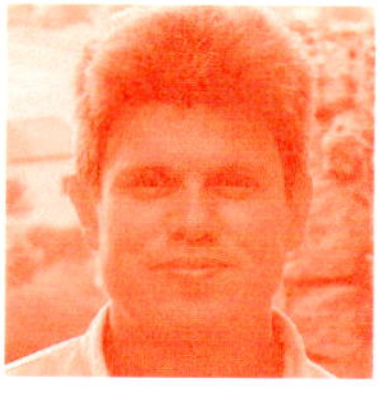

Robin Razmi is a resident physician at the Department of Infectious Diseases in Gävle Hospital, Sweden. He is interested in topics such as antibiotics, antimicrobial resistance, and disease control measures, and is active in the deployment of antibiotic stewardship at the hospital. He is affiliated to the Center for Research and Development Region Gävleborg, Uppsala University, Sweden. Dr. Razmi is very passionate about teaching, and strives to spread awareness about infectious diseases and the threat posed by emerging antimicrobial resistance.

Contents

Preface

Infective endocarditis is a potentially devastating disease. It presents with vague, unspecific symptoms, and both the suspicion and confirmation of the diagnosis is often delayed. The incidence of endocarditis has increased due to the aging population, with comorbidities, the vast use of implantable cardiac devices, artificial valves, and intravenous abuse. The diagnostic work-up relies on cardiac imaging, especially echocardiography and laboratory findings, in addition to careful history taking. A multidisciplinary team is warranted to achieve optimal treatment of patients with infectious endocarditis.

This book aims to cover various aspects of the management of infectious endocarditis. Hopefully, it may provide knowledge to implement improved, evidenced-based care for this challenging disease.

We hope you enjoy reading it!

Peter Magnusson (editor) and Robin Razmi (co-editor)
Peter Magnusson, MD
Centre for Research and Development, Uppsala University, Sweden,
Cardiology Research Unit, Department of Medicine, Karolinska Institutet,
Stockholm, Sweden

Robin Razmi
Centre for Research and Development, Uppsala University, Sweden

Chapter 1

Introductory Chapter: Infective Endocarditis - An Introduction

Robin Razmi and Peter Magnusson

1. Introduction

Infective endocarditis (IE) is a rare but potentially fatal condition. Almost always it is caused by bacteria, even though fungal endocarditis may occur. The infectious agent enters the bloodstream where it may adhere to the endocardium and predominantly the cardiac valves. While infective endocarditis (IE) may occur in any person, some risk factors are well known. Among these, the most significant are patients with valvular anomalies, prosthetic valves, cardiac implantable electric devices (CIEDs), and intravenous drug users. The clinical presentation may vary greatly depending on factors pertaining to the host as well as the causative microbe. Initial symptoms may be low-grade and unspecific but occasionally fulminant and severe. The diagnosis is often challenging and based on a combination of several clinical, microbiological, and radiological findings. The cornerstone of treatment is high-dose antibiotics, which are generally administered intravenously. However, pharmaceutical treatment alone is sometimes insufficient, and surgical intervention is required. This is particularly true in complicated cases, as well as in prosthetic valve endocarditis and CIED infection.

2. Epidemiology, pathophysiology, and prophylaxis

Bacteremia is a prerequisite for the development of infective endocarditis [1], and it is a more common phenomenon than might be assumed. In fact, transient bacteremia often occurs in various dental and surgical procedures, as well as in toothbrushing, flossing, and even chewing [2]. Despite the ubiquity of transient bacteremia, infective endocarditis is a rare condition with annual incidence in the USA varying between 11 and 15 cases per 100,000 population in the first 12 years of the new millennium [3]. It can thus be surmised that bacteremia alone is insufficient to cause the condition. Data from animal models suggest that the development of IE is dependent on the existence of a valvular lesion, which may be symptomatic, previously unknown or even microscopic, and clinically insignificant. The lesion in turn allows bacteria to adhere to the endocardial surface, promoting the establishment of the principal lesion in infective endocarditis: the vegetation [4].

The degree of valvular damage that is sufficient to cause disease varies greatly depending on the causative agent. *Staphylococcus aureus* has an exceptional status in this regard, owing to its recognized tendency to cause IE in patients without a pre-existing valvular condition. Infectious material in the bloodstream causes an upregulation of the body's inflammatory response. Fractions of the vegetation may come loose and cause embolization of other organs. Additionally, the presence of a vegetation on the endocardial surface may contribute irreversible structural damage [3].

The topic of antibiotic prophylaxis to prevent IE is a subject of controversy. As described above, transient bacteremia is very common in the general population,

IntechOpen

while manifest infective endocarditis is rare. Concordantly, striving to administer antibiotics to all individuals at risk for transient bacteremia would be a futile endeavor. Indications for prophylaxis in surgical and dental procedures have varied over the years, but it has never been proven that general prophylaxis is indicated, regardless of whether the procedure is high or low risk. Current recommendations, as put forward by the European Society of Cardiology, assert that antibiotic prophylaxis only be considered in high-risk procedures in patients with a pre-existing heart condition that confers a heightened risk of endocarditis. These include prosthetic valve, cyanotic congenital heart disease, and patients with a previous episode of IE. Antibiotic prophylaxis is not recommended in other forms of valvular or congenital heart disease [5].

3. Clinical symptoms, diagnosis, and imaging

Infective endocarditis is a condition whose presentation may vary greatly, which consequently may make the diagnosis elusive, conferring a significant delay in initiation of treatment. The presenting symptoms stem from several distinct pathophysiological mechanisms, and any combination of these may occur in any given individual:

- Symptoms of disseminated infection
- Symptoms of structural cardiac damage

Definite infective endocarditis
Pathologic criteria
1. Microorganisms demonstrated by culture or histologic examination of a vegetation, a vegetation that has embolized, or an intracardiac abscess specimen
2. Pathologic lesions; vegetation or intracardiac abscess confirmed by histologic examination
Showing active endocarditis
Clinical criteria
1. Two major criteria
2. One major criterion and three minor criteria
3. Five minor criteria
Possible infective endocarditis
1. One major criterion and one minor criterion
2. Three minor criteria
Rejected
1. Firm alternate diagnosis explaining evidence of infective endocarditis
2. Resolution of infective endocarditis syndrome with antibiotic therapy for < 4 days
3. No pathologic evidence of infective endocarditis at surgery or autopsy, with antibiotic therapy for <4 days
4. Does not meet criteria for possible infective endocarditis, as above

Table 1.
Modified Duke criteria [6].

- Symptoms of an upregulated immune system and circulating immune complexes

- Symptoms of septic embolism to distant organs

These mechanisms are reflected in the diagnostic criteria (the Duke criteria) provided in **Table 1** [6]. To accurately make an IE diagnosis, it is crucial to (a) perform a thorough clinical examination, (b) acquire adequate microbiological samples, and (c) ensure that correct radiological imaging is carried out. As to the latter, the cornerstone of radiological imaging has long been echocardiography: preferably with a transesophageal approach. Other modalities, such as ECG-triggered computerized tomography and positron emission tomography, are sometimes used in clinical practice, but are as yet not included in the Duke criteria [5].

4. Microbiology, antibiotic treatment, and surgery

The most common etiologic agents in IE are Gram-positive bacteria, which are responsible for more than 90% of cases. IE caused by Gram-negative bacteria and fungi does occur but rarely. While traditionally the major bacterial finding has been streptococcal species, later decades have seen a continuing rise of *S. aureus* [3].

Regardless of etiology, treatment consists of a long course of high-dose antibiotics, which are generally administered intravenously for the entire duration. Length of the treatment is usually 2–4 weeks but may be longer in complicated cases—particularly in those involving foreign material in the bloodstream. Due to the high total drug exposure, it is imperative to use pharmaceuticals which are well tolerated by the majority of patients. As in other severe infections, antibiotics of the beta-lactamase class are preferred when applicable. These drugs are distinguished by a combination of high efficacy and good tolerability [7].

Pharmaceutical treatment alone is often insufficient, however. Thoracic surgery is required in 25–50% of cases during acute infection and 20–40% during convalescence. Surgery is effective (a) as a means of source control (b) in preventing embolization and (c) as a means to repair structural cardiac damage [8]. Procedural risk is significant, however, and the decision to operate should be taken on an individual basis and in collaboration with representatives of appropriate clinical and diagnostic specialties. To this end it is recommended that decisions are taken by a unit known as the endocarditis team [9].

5. Conclusion

The aim of this book is to provide a deepened understanding of infective endocarditis which is a complex condition. Due to its diverse clinical features, patients with infective endocarditis may present at any part of the healthcare system, and awareness is crucial in order to establish a rapid and accurate diagnosis. In order to prevent mortality, as well as morbidity arising from embolic events and structural cardiac damage, it is important that appropriate medical and surgical management be initiated promptly in each individual case.

Author details

Robin Razmi[1] and Peter Magnusson[1,2]*

1 Centre for Research and Development, Uppsala University/Region Gävleborg, Sweden

2 Cardiology Research Unit, Department of Medicine, Karolinska Institute, Sweden

*Address all correspondence to: peter.magnusson@regiongavleborg.se

References

[1] Angrist AA, Oka M. Pathogenesis of bacterial endocarditis. *Journal of the American Medical Association*. 1963;**183**:249

[2] Simon GL. Transient bacteremia and endocarditis prophylaxis. *Archives of Internal Medicine*. 1984;**144**(1):34-35

[3] DeSimone D, Wilson W, Baddour L. Trends in infective endocarditis incidence, microbiology, and valve replacement in the United States from 2000 to 2011. *Journal of the American College of Cardiology*. 2015;**66**(10):1201-1202

[4] McGowan DA, Gillett R. Scanning electron microscopic observations of the surface of the initial lesion in experimental streptococcal endocarditis in the rabbit. *British Journal of Experimental Pathology*. 1980;**61**:164

[5] Habib G, Lancellotti P, Antunes MJ, et al. 2015 ESC guidelines for the management of infective endocarditis: The task force for the management of infective endocarditis of the European society of cardiology (ESC). Endorsed by: European association for cardio-thoracic surgery (EACTS), the European association of nuclear medicine (EANM). *European Heart Journal*. 2015;**36**(44):3075-3128

[6] Li J, Sexton D, Mick N, et al. Proposed modifications to the duke criteria for the diagnosis of infective endocarditis. Clinical Infectious Diseases. 2000;**30**(4):633-638

[7] Gould FK, Denning DW, Elliott TS, et al. Guidelines for the diagnosis and antibiotic treatment of endocarditis in adults: A report of the working party of the British society for antimicrobial chemotherapy. The Journal of Antimicrobial Chemotherapy. 2012;**67**:269-289

[8] Prendergast B, Tornos P. Surgery for infective endocarditis. *Circulation*. 2010;**121**(9):1141-1152

[9] Chambers J, Sandoe J, Ray S, et al. The infective endocarditis team: Recommendations from an international working group. *Heart*. 2014;**100**:524-527

Chapter 2

Right-Sided Infective Endocarditis Secondary to Intravenous Drug Abuse

Ruchika Meel

Abstract

Right-sided infective endocarditis is due to intravenous drug abuse. Right-sided infective endocarditis is rare. It comprises 5–10% of infective endocarditis cases. Traditionally, it has been reported more commonly in patients with medical devices such as pacemakers and defibrillators and dialysis catheters. Recently, there has been increase in right-sided infective endocarditis related to intravenous drug abuse. Right-sided infective endocarditis related to drug abuse mostly affects the tricuspid valve and rarely the pulmonary valve. Although, most uncomplicated cases do well with medical treatment, it is associated with considerable morbidity and mortality due to recurrent infection. Surgery for right-sided infective endocarditis is uncommon especially in resource limited setting. Few current studies have explored surgical options in this group of patients. This chapter will review current literature related to right-sided infective endocarditis due to intravenous drug abuse.

Keywords: infective endocarditis, intravenous drug abuse

1. Introduction

Infective endocarditis (IE) is characterised by a microbial infection that involves the endocardial surface of the heart; it most often denotes infection of the heart valves or an intracardiac device [1]. Less commonly it involves septal defects, mural endocardium and the subvalvular apparatus [2]. The classic lesion is a vegetation, which is composed of platelets, fibrin enmeshed with microorganisms and inflammatory cells [3]. Infective endocarditis is caused by many different species of bacteria such as staphylococci, streptococci, enterococci and slow-growing Gram-negative coccobacilli.

In the 1950s IE secondary to intravenous drug use was first described [4]. Right-sided infective endocarditis (RSIE) secondary to intravenous drug use is a distinct entity and will be reviewed in this chapter.

2. Epidemiology

Intravenous drug abuse (IVDA) is a recognised risk factor for IE. Intravenous drug users are at a seven times higher risk for infective endocarditis compared to patients with rheumatic heart disease or prosthetic valves [3].

Over the last decade there has been a steady increase in number of cases related to IE due to intravenous drug use. Between 2000 and 2008 the rate of IE due to IVDA has increased from 6 to 8% hospitalisation to 12% in the year 2013. During this period there has been an increase in IVDA related IE cases amongst younger white population. A similar distribution was noted between males and females [5].

In United States, North Carolina, a study reported a 12-fold increase in hospitalisations for intravenous drug use related IE over the last decade [6].

In the past IE related to IVDA was predominantly disease of men. A recent study has shown that there is a general increase in the rate of IVDA associated IE in the United States, with a relatively higher proportion of women compared to previous studies [5, 6]. In a recent South African Study, Meel et al. reported an increase in the incidence of IE related to IVDA amongst Africans. These were predominantly male and majority were HIV infected [7].

Infective endocarditis involving the right side accounts for 5–10% of cases of IE [8, 9].

RSIE may occur in patients with intracardiac devices but in intravenous drug users it is usually associated with HIV infection [9].

HIV infection in intravenous drug users is associated with a higher rate of IE compared to HIV uninfected users [10, 11]. Further, immunosuppression with lower CD4 count is associated with a higher predisposition to IE [9].

Intravenous drug use related IE involves the tricuspid valve in 46–78% of the cases, mitral valve in 24–32% of cases and the aortic valve in 8–19%. About 16% of the patients have multiple valve involvement. In the majority the infection occurs on the native valves. Intravenous drug use is characterised by recurrent infective endocarditis of the native valves [3].

3. Etiopathogenesis

The most common organism isolated in IVDA related IE is *Staphylococcus aureus*. It accounts for greater than 50% of the organisms cultured [3]. It tends to commonly infect the native tricuspid valve. In contrast streptococci and enterococci infect damaged valves, mostly aortic and the mitral valve. Other organisms include fungi, *Pseudomonas aeruginosa* and Gram-negative bacilli. Injection of contaminated material predisposes drug addicts to less commonly encountered organisms such as *Corynebacterium* species, *Lactobacillus*, *Neisseria* species and *Bacillus cereus*. In 3–5% of cases Polymicrobial infection is present [3].

The tricuspid valve is the most commonly involved valve in RSIE due to IVDA. Injection of recreational drugs results in entry of particulate matter such as talc into the circulatory system resulting in structural damage to the endothelium of the valve [12, 13]. Similarly, the left-sided valves get damaged by particulate matter that is less than 10 mm in size and is able to cross the pulmonary circulation [14]. The use of cocaine is associated with greater frequency of IE in IVDA. The possible mechanisms postulated include the ability of cocaine to cause vasospasm and tissue damage to the myocardium. It is also procoagulant and thus can cause thrombus formation and thus producing a nidus for bacterial seeding the damaged valve tissue [8]. Further, it has been postulated that intravenous drugs can result in pulmonary hypertension leading to increased turbulent blood flow across the valve resulting in endothelial damage to the right-sided heart valves.

The pathogenesis of formation of vegetation is complex. It involves interaction between the host, the organism, the endothelium, hemostatic pathways, the ability of the hosts immune system to eliminate the organism and the virulence of the specific microorganism [3].

The microorganism once in the blood stream tend to attach themselves to the valve surface and proliferate at sites of endothelial damage resulting in further damage to the valve tissue. The microorganisms initially attach to the platelet-fibrin nidus and then proliferate [15]. Microbial growth results in activation of the extrinsic coagulation pathway, monocytes release a myriad of pro-inflammatory cytokines and there is increased expression of fibronectin on the surface of the endothelial cells with resultant formation of a vegetation.

The vegetation grows further, with subsequent embolization and continued bacteraemia, if the host is unable to contain the infection [16].

4. Clinical features

Right-sided infective endocarditis usually presents with fever, persistent bacteraemia and septic emboli to the lungs. Initial presentation may comprise haemoptysis, cough or chest pain. Peripheral embolization must alert one to the presence of concomitant left-sided endocarditis or a shunt. Right heart failure is a result of both pressure and volume overload from pulmonary hypertension or organic tricuspid regurgitation or rarely obstruction of the tricuspid orifice by a vegetation [17, 18].

Pulmonary septic emboli may be complicated by pulmonary infarction, abscess, pneumothorax, and purulent pulmonary effusion [17] (**Figures 1** and **2**).

It is important to note that patients with RSIE do not always have an audible murmur of tricuspid regurgitation [13]. Other features unique to this group of patients with IE are the presence of co-infections with HIV, hepatitis C and hepatitis B infections, which complicate their clinical management and adversely affect their outcomes. A high degree of suspicion of IE must be maintained in IVDA as their clinical assessment can be quite challenging, especially in those who do not manifest the classic clinical features.

Additionally, the sensitivity and specificity of the modified Duke's criteria in right-sided endocarditis has not been studied. Inclusion of septic pulmonary infarcts as a minor criteria in the modified Duke's criteria may therefore be inappropriate [19].

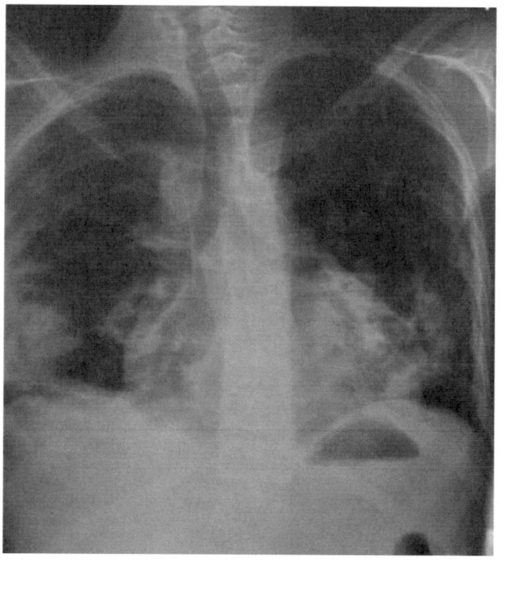

Figure 1.
An anterior-posterior chest X-ray showing increased cardiothoracic index with areas of alveolar opacification involving both lung fields likely representing septic embolization and abscess formation in the lungs.

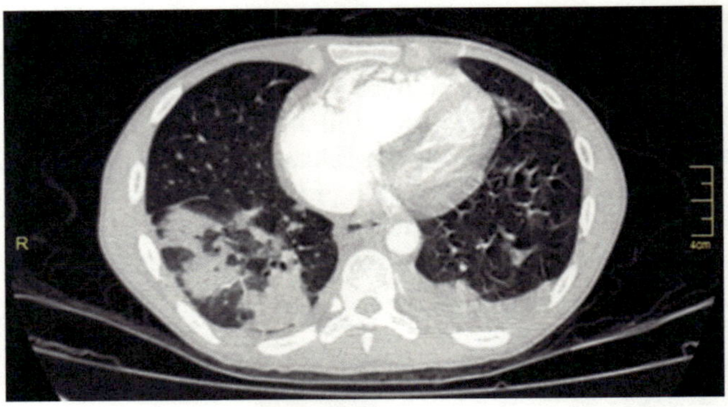

Figure 2.
Multiple areas of consolidation suggestive of infarction and dilated right heart chambers on a CT scan of the chest of a patient with history of right-sided infective endocarditis due to intravenous drug abuse.

5. Diagnosis

In addition to the above mentioned clinical features and positive blood cultures, transthoracic echocardiography (TTE) greatly aids in establishing a diagnosis of IE,

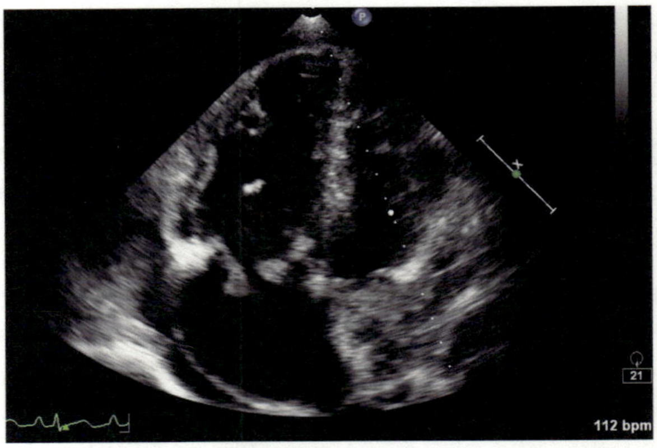

Figure 3.
Modified apical four-chamber view showing multiple vegetations on the tricuspid valve (arrow) with a dilated right atrium and right ventricle.

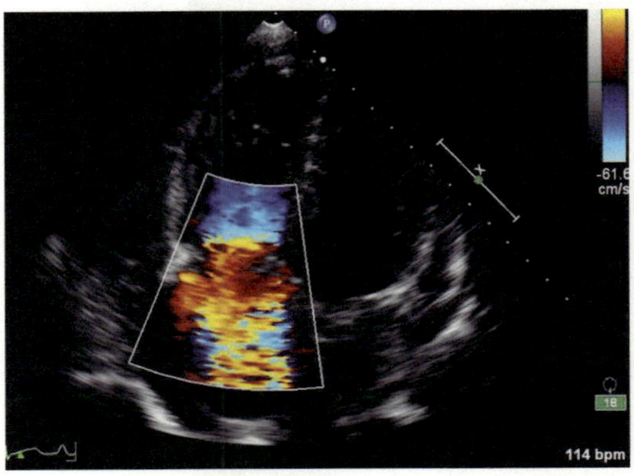

Figure 4.
Colour Doppler ultrasound showing severe tricuspid regurgitation.

especially in cases with equivocal clinical presentation. TTE allows easy visualisation of vegetations on the anteriorly located tricuspid valve and associated tricuspid regurgitation (**Figures 3** and **4**) [20, 21].

A transesophageal echocardiography may be required in detection of vegetations on the pulmonary valve and for exclusion of left-sided valve involvement [22]. The Eustachian valve must be screened for presence of vegetations.

6. Management

The initial antimicrobial therapy should take into account four factors: (1) suspected organism (2) type of drug (3) the solvent used by the addict and (4) the location of Infection [17].

Empirical therapy in acute severely ill patients must consist of ampicillin and cloxacillin with gentamycin or vancomycin with gentamycin (in patients allergic to penicillin) [17]. *Staphylococcus aureus* must always be covered. Anti-pseudomonas agent must be added in a pentazocine drug addict. If an IVDA gives a history of brown heroin use mixed with lemon juice then an anti-fungal agent must be added due to a high risk of candida septicaemia. Anti-microbial therapy can be de-escalated once the specific causative organism is isolated on blood cultures.

Due to reluctance of IVDA for prolonged hospital admission and the concerns related to their discharge on intravenous antibiotic therapy, a few studies have studied the possibility of treating IE in these patients with short course antibiotic therapy [23].

A 2 week treatment regimen has been advocated in non-complicated isolated tricuspid valve endocarditis. These patients must have low risk features such as good response to therapy, methicillin sensitive *Staphylococcus aureus*, small vegetation size (less than 20 mm), no features of peripheral embolization, absence of metastatic infection, lack of involvement of left-sided valves or prosthetic valve and absence of a severely immunosuppressed state. In such cases, a short 2 week course of intravenous cloxacillin or oxacillin alone may be used [24]. These patients must be closely followed up and the response to therapy must be assessed.

In complicated cases a 4–6 week course of intravenous therapy must be utilised. These include situations where there is poor response to antibiotic therapy, large vegetation size (>20 mm), septic emboli, use of penicillinase non-resistant antibiotics, and a severely immunosuppressed state such as HIV with a CD4 count less than 200cell/ml and associated involvement of left-sided valves [25–27].

Due to a high rate of recurrent IE in IVDA, surgery should only be considered in the following situations: (1) intractable right-sided heart failure with poor response to diuretics; (2) persistent bacteraemia despite use of appropriate antimicrobial therapy; and (3) large vegetation size of greater than 20 mm that do not diminish in size after repeated episodes of pulmonary emboli [25, 28, 29].

In general the outcomes of patients with IVDA related IE have been poor post surgery. A substantially high long term mortality has been reported for IE related surgery in IVDA compared to non-drug users [30–32].

In HIV-infected IVDAs with IE cardiac surgery does not worsen the outcome of either the IE or the HIV [17]. Patients with advanced HIV infection with severe immunosuppression. However, valve replacement surgery may have unacceptably high risks in selected patients with advanced HIV infection, low CD4 counts, and either a history of failed antiretroviral therapy or ongoing drug abuse that precludes therapy with antiretroviral agents [33].

The most commonly performed surgery for tricuspid valve endocarditis includes valvectomy, valve replacement or repair [34]. Valve repair is advocated by some studies but repair has not proven to be superior to either valve replacement or valvectomy. In a few cases of RSIE valvectomy may be performed initially followed by subsequent bioprosthetic valve replacement once the infection has subsided and drug use discontinued. Pulmonary valve rarely requires replacement except in extreme cases of valve destruction. In cases where pulmonary valve replacement is deemed suitable, a homograft is preferred.

7. Prognosis

Overall, IVDA with RSIE have a lower mortality than those with left-sided infective endocarditis [14, 24, 35–39]. In one study the mortality was noted to be 6% [40]. Factors associated with high mortality included a large vegetation size (>20 mm) and a fungal aetiology [41, 42].

In general patients with HIV do not have a poor outcome, except those with CD4 count <200 cells/ml. The major reason for repeat hospitalisation and recurrent endocarditis in IVDA is related to persistent use of drugs [30, 43, 44].

Finally, management of RSIE related to IVDA poses some ethical dilemmas. From the limited available literature, surgery should be offered for patients with surgical indications, with a first episode of IE in IVDAs, who are willing to undergo rehabilitation. If the patient presents with a second episode of IE due to recurrent IVDA, the decision to re-operate the patient, if indicated, is complex. It should be individualised and discussed by the endocarditis team. It is reasonable to decline further surgical intervention in this group, especially in resource-limited settings [45].

Author details

Ruchika Meel
Division of Cardiology, Chris Hani Baragwanath Academic Hospital and University of the Witwatersrand, Johannesburg, South Africa

*Address all correspondence to: ruchikameel@gmail.com

References

[1] Sexton DJ, Fowler VG. Clinical manifestations and evaluation of adults with suspected native valve endocarditis. U: UpToDate. Otto CM, ur., Baron EL, ur. UpToDate (Internet). 2017:1-50

[2] Mylonakis E, Calderwood SB. Infective endocarditis in adults. New England Journal of Medicine. 2001;**345**:1318-1330

[3] Lilly LS, Braunwald E. Braunwald's Heart Disease: A Textbook of Cardiovascular Medicine. Philadelphia: Elsevier Health Sciences; 2012

[4] Hussey HH, Katz S. Infections resulting from narcotic addiction; report of 102 cases. The American Journal of Medicine. 1950;**9**:186

[5] Wurcel AG, Anderson JE, Chui KK, et al. Increasing infectious endocarditis admissions among young people who inject drugs. Open Forum Infectious Diseases. 2016;**3**:ofw157

[6] Schranz AJ, Fleischauer A, Chu VH, et al. Trends in drug use-associated infective endocarditis and heart valve surgery, 2007 to 2017: A study of Statewide discharge data. Annals of Internal Medicine. 2019;**170**:31-40

[7] Meel R, Essop M. Striking increase in the incidence of infective endocarditis associated with recreational drug abuse in urban South Africa. South African Medical Journal. 2018;**108**(7):585-589

[8] Frontera JA, Gradon JD. Right-side endocarditis in injection drug users: Review of proposed mechanisms of pathogenesis. Clinical Infectious Diseases. 2000;**30**:374-379

[9] Wilson LE, Thomas DL, Astemborski J, Freedman TL, Vlahov D. Prospective study of infective endocarditis among injection drug users. The Journal of Infectious Diseases. 2002;**185**:1761-1766

[10] Spijkerman IJ, van Ameijden EJ, Mientjes GH, et al. Human immunodeficiency virus infection and other risk factors for skin abscesses and endocarditis among injection drug users. Journal of Clinical Epidemiology. 1996;**49**:1149

[11] Manoff SB, Vlahov D, Herskowitz A, et al. Human immunodeficiency virus infection and infective endocarditis among injecting drug users. Epidemiology. 1996;**7**:566

[12] Weinstein WL, Brusch JL. Infective Endocarditis. New York City: Oxford University Press; 1996

[13] Sande MA, Lee BL, Mills J, et al. Endocarditis in intravenous drug users. In: Kaye D, editor. Infective Endocarditis. New York City: Raven Press; 1992. p. 345

[14] Mathew J, Addai T, Anand A, et al. Clinical features, site of involvement, bacteriologic findings, and outcome of infective endocarditis in intravenous drug users. Archives of Internal Medicine. 1995;**155**:1641

[15] Durack DT, Beeson PB. Experimental bacterial endocarditis. I. Colonization of a sterile vegetation. British Journal of Experimental Pathology. 1972;**53**:44

[16] Werdan K, Dietz S, Löffler B, et al. Mechanisms of infective endocarditis: Pathogen-host interaction and risk states. Nature Reviews. Cardiology. 2014;**11**:35

[17] Habib G, Lancellotti P, Antunes MJ, Bongiorni MG, Casalta JP, Del Zotti F, Dulgheru R, El Khoury G, Erba PA, Iung B, Miro JM. 2015 ESC guidelines for the management of infective endocarditis: The task force for the management of infective endocarditis of the European Society of Cardiology (ESC)

endorsed by: European Association for Cardio-Thoracic Surgery (EACTS), the European Association of Nuclear Medicine (EANM). European Heart Journal. 2015;**36**:3075-3128

[18] Carozza A, De Santo LS, Romano G, Della CA, Ursomando F, Scardone M, et al. Infective endocarditis in intravenous drug abusers: Patterns of presentation and long-term outcomes of surgical treatment. The Journal of Heart Valve Disease. 2006;**15**:125-131

[19] Westphal N, Plicht B, Naber C. Infective endocarditis—Prophylaxis, diagnostic criteria, and treatment. Deutsches Ärzteblatt International. 2009;**106**(28-29):481

[20] San Roman JA, Vilacosta I, Lopez J, Revilla A, Arnold R, Sevilla T, et al. Role of transthoracic and transesophageal echocardiography in right-sided endocarditis: One echocardiographic modality does not fit all. Journal of the American Society of Echocardiography. 2012;**25**:807-814

[21] San Roman JA, Vilacosta I, Zamorano JL, Almeria C, Sanchez-Harguindey L. Transesophageal echocardiography in right-sided endocarditis. Journal of the American College of Cardiology. 1993;**21**:1226-1230

[22] Winslow T, Foster E, Adams JR, Schiller NB. Pulmonary valve endocarditis: Improveddiagnosis with biplane transesophageal echocardiography. Journal of the American Society of Echocardiography. 1992;**5**:206-210

[23] Suzuki J, Johnson J, Montgomery M, et al. Outpatient parenteral antimicrobial therapy among people who inject drugs: A review of the literature. Open Forum Infectious Diseases. 2018;**5**:ofy194

[24] Ribera E, Gomez-Jimenez J, Cortes E, del Valle O, Planes A, Gonzalez-Alujas T, et al. Effectiveness of cloxacillin with and without gentamicin in short-term therapy for right-sided *Staphylococcus aureus* endocarditis. A randomized, controlled trial. Annals of Internal Medicine. 1996;**125**:969-974

[25] Hecht SR, Berger M. Right-sided endocarditis in intravenous drug users. Prognostic features in 102 episodes. Annals of Internal Medicine. 1992;**117**:560-566

[26] Fortun J, Pérez-Molina JA, Añón MT, Martinez-Beltran J, Loza E, Guerrero A. Right-sided endocarditis caused by *Staphylococcus aureus* in drug abusers. Antimicrobial Agents and Chemotherapy. 1995;**39**:525-528

[27] Pulvirenti JJ, Kerns E, Benson C, Lisowski J, Demarais P, Weinstein RA. Infective endocarditis in injection drug users: Importance of human immunodeficiency virus serostatus and degree of immunosuppression. Clinical Infectious Diseases. 1996;**22**:40-45

[28] Akinosoglou K, Apostolakis E, Koutsogiannis N, Leivaditis V, Gogos CA. Rightsided infective endocarditis: Surgical management. European Journal of Cardio-Thoracic Surgery 2012;**42**:470-479

[29] Botsford KB, Weinstein RA, Nathan CR, Kabins SA. Selective survival in pentazocine and tripelennamine of *Pseudomonas aeruginosa* serotype O11 from drug addicts. The Journal of Infectious Diseases. 1985;**151**:209-216

[30] Rabkin DG, Mokadam NA, Miller DW, et al. Long-term outcome for the surgical treatment of infective endocarditis with a focus on intravenous drug users. The Annals of Thoracic Surgery. 2012;**93**:51

[31] Thalme A, Westling K, Julander I. In-hospital and long-term mortality in infective endocarditis in injecting drug users compared to non-drug users:

A retrospective study of 192 episodes. Scandinavian Journal of Infectious Diseases. 2007;**39**:197

[32] Kim JB, Ejiofor JI, Yammine M, et al. Surgical outcomes of infective endocarditis among intravenous drug users. The Journal of Thoracic and Cardiovascular Surgery. 2016;**152**:832

[33] Sexton DJ, Chu VH. Epidemiology, Risk Factors and Microbiology of Infective Endocarditis. Waltham: UpToDate; 2011

[34] Gaca JG, Sheng S, Daneshmand M, Rankin JS, Williams ML, O'Brien SM, et al. Current outcomes for tricuspid valve infective endocarditis surgery in North America. The Annals of Thoracic Surgery. 2013;**96**:1374-1381

[35] Ortiz-Bautista C, López J, García-Granja PE, et al. Current profile of infective endocarditis in intravenous drug users: The prognostic relevance of the valves involved. International Journal of Cardiology. 2015;**187**:472

[36] Abrams B, Sklaver A, Hoffman T, Greenman R. Single or combination therapy of staphylococcal endocarditis in intravenous drug abusers. Annals of Internal Medicine. 1979;**90**:789

[37] Menda KB, Gorbach SL. Favorable experience with bacterial endocarditis in heroin addicts. Annals of Internal Medicine. 1973;**78**:25

[38] DiNubile MJ. Short-course antibiotic therapy for right-sided endocarditis caused by *Staphylococcus aureus* in injection drug users. Annals of Internal Medicine. 1994;**121**:873

[39] Mathew J, Abreo G, Namburi K, et al. Results of surgical treatment for infective endocarditis in intravenous drug users. Chest. 1995;**108**:73

[40] Martín-Dávila P, Navas E, Fortún J, et al. Analysis of mortality and risk factors associated with native valve endocarditis in drug users: The importance of vegetation size. American Heart Journal. 2005;**150**:1099

[41] Robbins MJ, Frater RW, Soeiro R, et al. Influence of vegetation size on clinical outcome of right-sided infective endocarditis. The American Journal of Medicine. 1986;**80**:165

[42] Bayer AS, Blomquist IK, Bello E, et al. Tricuspid valve endocarditis due to *Staphylococcus aureus*. Correlation of two-dimensional echocardiography with clinical outcome. Chest. 1988;**93**:247

[43] Østerdal OB, Salminen PR, Jordal S, et al. Cardiac surgery for infective endocarditis in patients with intravenous drug use. Interactive Cardiovascular and Thoracic Surgery. 2016;**22**:633

[44] Rosenthal ES, Karchmer AW, Theisen-Toupal J, et al. Suboptimal addiction interventions for patients hospitalized with injection drug use-associated infective endocarditis. The American Journal of Medicine. 2016;**129**:481

[45] Yeo KK, Chang WS, Lau JM, et al. Valve replacement in endocarditis: Setting limits in noncompliant intravenous drug abusers. Hawaii Medical Journal. 2006;**65**:168-171

Chapter 3

Right-Sided Infective Endocarditis

Adrian Fernando Narvaez Muñoz and Daniela Albina Ibarra Vargas

Abstract

Infective endocarditis (IE) at the right side represents the 5–10% of IE cases. It is more frequent in people with intravenous drug addiction (IVDA); however, there is another population susceptible to this infection; hemodialytic patients, intracardiac devices, and congenital heart diseases are included inside this group. Right-sided infective endocarditis (RSIE) has lower mortality than the left-sided infective endocarditis (LSIE). Common symptoms secondary to right-sided endocarditis are the respiratory symptoms characterized by a cough, hemoptysis, persistent fever, dyspnea, and chest pain. Echocardiography and blood cultures are the first tools to perform the diagnosis. The tricuspid valve is the main anatomical structure affected. Medical treatment with antibiotic therapy resolves the infection majority of the time; the surgical treatment is indicated in some cases, such as right-heart failure due to severe tricuspid valve regurgitation; inability to eliminate bacteremia or organism; resistance to culture-directed antibiotic treatment, within 7 days; and tricuspid valve vegetations >20 mm. RSIE implies a better prognosis than LSIE. Concomitant left-sided IE carries a worse prognosis than right-sided infection alone, due predominantly to its greater likelihood for invasion and abscess formation.

Keywords: infective endocarditis, right-sided infective endocarditis, tricuspid valve, intravenous drug addiction, echocardiography, antibiotic, surgery, hemodialysis, intensive care unit, pulmonary valve

1. Introduction

Infective endocarditis (IE) at the right side of the heart is quite rare; it represents the 5–10% of IE cases. It is seen most frequently in people with intravenous drug addiction; nevertheless, other portions of the population are in high risk of developing this disease such as patients with indwelling catheters, cardiac devices, congenital cardiac pathologies, and immunocompromised diseases [1–3].

The evolution of right-heart IE is much better than the left-side IE with a lower rate of mortality (3–30%) [3]. This pathology is more frequent in people between 20 and 61 years, with a mean age of 38 $\pm$ 15 years [4].

Staphylococcus aureus is the predominant organism (60–90% of cases) with the methicillin-resistant strains becoming more prevalent lately [3, 5]. The tricuspid valve is by far the most effective structure (90%) in right-side infective endocarditis (RSIE) [5].

2. Diagnosis

2.1 Clinic manifestations

Common symptoms secondary to right-sided endocarditis are the respiratory symptoms characterized by a cough, hemoptysis, persistent fever, dyspnea, and chest pain [4].

In exceptional circumstances, right-heart failure can arise, generated by the increase in pulmonary pressure, severe tricuspid valve regurgitation, or obstruction of pulmonary circulation through multiple pulmonary emboli [4, 6].

The diagnosis of RSIE is often delayed because the signs and symptoms are relatively different concerning the LSIE clinical setting; the Duke's modified criteria do not have value in the RSIE. The low incidence of RSIE also plays an essential factor in the underdiagnosis of this disease.

There are reports in which the 76% of the patients had gotten an antibacterial treatment before the endocarditis's diagnosis because they developed some signs and symptoms that were misunderstood as a febrile syndrome or pneumonia [4].

An acute beginning of the disease is seen at the majority of the patients; only a few cases have been reported with chronic symptoms (more of 2 months) [4].

It is frequent that right-side vegetations dislodge microemboli to the pulmonary region. The pulmonary embolism (PE) can induce pulmonary infarction, abscesses, pneumothoraxes, and purulent pulmonary effusions.

Persistent fever associated with pulmonary events, anemia, and microscopic hematuria, the so-called "tricuspid syndrome," is the sign of clinical alert for tricuspid valve IE [3, 4, 7].

Revilla et al. found 24% of their patients with this syndrome, and the other 65% had at least two of the three signs [4].

2.2 Complementary exams

2.2.1 Laboratory

Nowadays it is routinary to order blood tests for any patient admitted at the hospital, and it is reasonably used if the suspicion of infection is thought. Some findings such as high titers of white blood cells, procalcitonin, and C-reactive protein can support the infection diagnosis; nevertheless, these variables are not used as criteria to diagnose infective endocarditis [5, 8].

The anemia has been described as part of the tricuspid syndrome, so the values of hemoglobin and hematocrit below the normal range can be found in the blood test, which probably will reveal a normocytic, normochromic anemia patron [3, 4, 7].

The urine test can show microhematuria which also is part of the tricuspid syndrome.

2.2.2 Cultures

Right-sided endocarditis in IVDA is commonly caused by *S. aureus* and *Pseudomonas aeruginosa*, and other Gram-negative organisms, fungi, streptococci, and enterococci have also been found [4, 6].

In the majority of patients, the microorganism can be identified through blood cultures if they are adequately collected. The 2015 ESC endocarditis guidelines recommend a technique of recollection minutely sterile of at least three sets of samples with an interval of 30 minutes; each sample must contain 10 ml of blood and should be incubated in both aerobic and anaerobic atmospheres. Another crucial aspect is the recollection of samples from a peripheral vein instead of central venous catheter due to the risk of contamination and wrong interpretation [5].

Occasionally, the blood cultures can be negative by different reasons, especially if an antimicrobial therapy was established before the acquisition of the samples. The blood cultures usually become negatives after 48 hours from the beginning of antibiotics [4].

2.2.3 Image

Currently, the diagnosis of IE requires the finding of an infective process inside the heart, reason why the imaging techniques are valuable to diagnose or discard IE. The echocardiography is the most important and more used tool to diagnose, manage, and monitor patients with IE [5].

However, other imaging methods have been developed in the last decades, allowing us to back the diagnosis of IE when the echography is not entirely clear in some cases (**Table 1**).

2.2.3.1 Radiography

It can be quite normal or shows a variety of findings, such as cardiomegaly, pulmonary septic emboli, or pleural effusion [4].

2.2.3.2 Echocardiography

The benefits that the echocardiography brought to the cardiology area are well-known, and they can help us to detect anomalies related to IE. It is the gold standard imaging test for IE, becoming one of the first steps that we must do if IE is suspected [3, 9].

The same as the LSIE, the transthoracic echocardiography (TTE) is the first modality recommended to perform if RSIE is suspected. The sensitivity of TTE to detect vegetations is roughly 75% and its specificity over 90%. When the hunch of IE is high, but the TTE is negative, the transesophageal echocardiography (TOE) must be used because its sensitivity is higher than TTE, approximately 96%. Some experts indeed recommend TOE even if the TTE is positive for IE; nevertheless, it does not apply for RSIE in which an explicit finding of IE is enough for the diagnosis [5, 9].

Chest radiography	Echocardiography	Computed Tomography	Nuclear imaging
Cardiomegaly	Vegetations	Abscess	Cardiac enhancement
Pulmonary septic emboli	Abscess	Pseudoaneurysm	Septic emboli
Pleural effusion	Prosthetic dehiscence	Fistula	

Table 1.
Imaging technique findings in the right-sided infective endocarditis.

The 2015 ESC guidelines also suggest the use of TOE when the suspicion of IE is present in patients with a prosthetic heart valve and intracardiac device [5].

There are some "typical lesions" of IE that we can detect in the echocardiography, such as vegetations, abscess, pseudoaneurysm, valve aneurysm, perforation, fistula, and dehiscence of the prosthetic valve, being the vegetation of the landmark lesion of this disease (**Figure 1**) [5, 9].

Occasionally, parts of the vegetations can be visualized floating in the right ventricle or entrapped in the subvalvular apparatus. TTE usually allows assessment of tricuspid valve involvement because of the valve's anterior location and large natural vegetations. TOE imaging is more sensitive to detect vegetations than TTE imaging, especially in the case of abscesses, and associated left-sided involvement [6].

2.2.3.3 Computed tomography (CT)

Cardiac computed tomography (CCT) can improve the diagnosis of IE when abscesses and pseudoaneurysm are present, due to its higher sensitivity (approximately 81%) in comparison with TTE and TOE (roughly 63%). The combination of echocardiography and CCT to diagnose abscess/pseudoaneurysm reaches 100% sensitivity. In pulmonary/right-sided endocarditis, CT may reveal concomitant pulmonary disease, including abscesses and infarcts [5, 10].

2.2.3.4 Magnetic resonance (MR)

The use of MR in the IE setting is focused on the diagnosis of cerebrovascular events related to IE. This imaging modality has better sensitivity than CT to detect brain hemorrhage and infectious intracranial aneurysms (IIAs) [5, 11].

2.2.3.5 Nuclear imaging

The incorporation of positron-emission tomography (PET) in the modified Duke's criteria is addressed to enhance the IE diagnosis in some situations where the

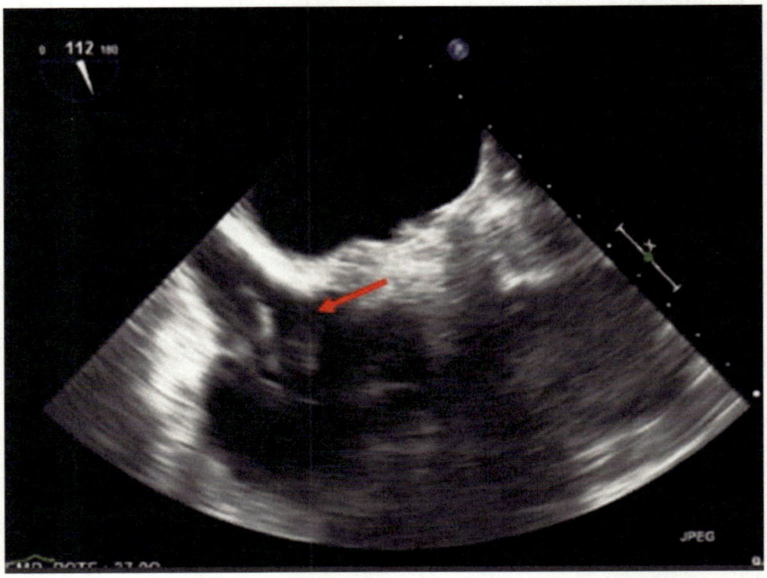

Figure 1.
Transesophageal echocardiogram: a hyperechoic lesion (red arrow) is seen at level of pulmonary valve, prolapsing to right ventricle outflow tract.

clinical suspicion is not always confirmed with the echocardiography. This imaging technique is especially valuable in the diagnosis of prosthetic valve infective endocarditis (PVIE) [5, 12].

There are also reports where the PET helped to determine the extension of pacemaker or defibrillator infection, consequently improving the adequate surgical intervention [13].

Peripheral embolic and metastatic infectious events can also be detected with this technique; nevertheless, their specificity is lower in brain septic emboli [5].

A correct interpretation of PET must be taken in some conditions which can make us misinterpret the findings, for instance, a recent cardiac surgery usually shows enhancement at the mediastinal area due to the inflammatory response. Some conditions can show similar patterns to that of IE, such as an active thrombus, soft atherosclerotic plaques, vasculitis, primary cardiac tumors, cardiac metastasis from a non-cardiac tumor, postsurgical inflammation, and foreign body reactions [5].

3. Treatment

3.1 Medical treatment

The same fundamental aspects about the antibiotic therapy in IE is applied to the right-sided endocarditis, making emphasis in the early and proper setting of the cultures, the prompt and adequate starting of empirical antimicrobial therapy (if the suspicious of IE is higher), and the administration of a culture-antibiogram sensible antibiotic.

One aspect that changed in the antimicrobial treatment of RSIE in comparison with LSIE is the duration of the therapy when the implicated bacteria is the methicillin-sensible *Staphylococcus aureus*, due to the 2015 European Society of Cardiology guidelines for the management of infective endocarditis recommending a short treatment of 2 weeks in this scenario. This approach is attributed to the less aggressive evolution of RSIE with these bacteria [5].

The prophylactic treatment in the patient with high suspicion of RSIE should cover *Staphylococcus aureus*, streptococci, and enterococci and should include penicillinase-resistant penicillins or vancomycin, depending on the local prevalence of methicillin-resistant *Staphylococcus aureus* (MRSA) [6].

3.2 Surgery treatment

In RSIE, the medical treatment usually resolves the disease; nevertheless, the surgery for right-sided infective endocarditis is recommended in the following situations: (1) right-heart failure due to severe tricuspid valve regurgitation, (2) inability to eliminate bacteremia or organisms resistant to culture-directed antibiotic treatment, within 7 days, and (3) tricuspid valve vegetations >20 mm [1–3, 5].

During the surgery, most of the infected tissue must be removed; if it is possible, we should try to repair the native valve but guarantee the adequate functioning of the valve. When a valve-sparing is impossible, the implantation of a prosthetic valve is necessary, always trying to use the less foreign material to diminish the risk of IE recurrence [14].

Sometimes the endocardial destruction is highly extensive that compromises the valve repairing as well as the valve prosthesis replacement; this scenario is hideous and requires the reconstruction of the annular structure using endocardium patch or other materials.

Another potential complication of IE can be the formation of ventricular septal defect due to the infection's aggressiveness which can show communication between the right ventricle and left ventricle through the membranous septum. This anatomical defect also can be figured out with a pericardium patch [15].

Some surgeons can feel uncomfortable with the idea of setting up a prosthetic valve in tricuspid position due to being afraid of high gradients through the valve and the potential thrombosis of the prosthesis. However, large prostheses (>30 mm) guarantee low transvalvular gradients, and the incidence of thrombosis is small if the patient has an adequate anticoagulation control (biological and mechanic prostheses are anticoagulated). Moreover, bioprosthesis degeneration develops more slowly owing to the low-pressure conditions in the right ventricle [6].

In 1991, Arbulu et al. published a paper showing their experience in tricuspid valvulectomy without replacement, generally indicated for IVDA, to avoid the potential IE recurrence; nevertheless, about 25% of patients cannot tolerate tricuspid regurgitation and require a second operation for tricuspid valve replacement [14, 16].

4. Prognosis

RSIE implies a better prognosis than LSIE; the previous study revealed the mortality of right-sided IE is 12% in-hospital patients and 0–7.3% for surgical patients. However, these percentages increase at least twice in patients with intensive care unit (ICU) admission; actually, this issue will be described forward [3, 9].

Concomitant left-sided IE carries a worse prognosis than right-sided infection alone, due predominantly to its greater likelihood for invasion and abscess formation [7].

5. Prevention

The high increase of bacterial resistance throughout the last decades has produced a change in the IE guidelines from 2002. The same criteria for LSIE are applied to RSIE regarding the antimicrobial prophylaxis, being reserved only in patients with a high risk of endocarditis, particularly those with PVIE [5].

Nevertheless, there are some aspects that the last IE guidelines do not approach which are very relevant that need to be highlighted. One of the most critical issues is the quite strict aseptic measurements that healthcare professionals must take during routine procedures, especially invasive maneuvers in high-risk patients such as immunocompromised, hemodialytic (HD), cyanotic congenital heart disease (CHD) patients, etc.

The change in some hospital policies can diminish the incidence of bacteremia and IE, such as have been shown in some publications [17].

6. RSIE in intensive care units (ICU)

There are few publications about the characteristics of RSIE in ICU. It is noteworthy that patients with IE admitted in ICU have a higher rate of morbidity and mortality than non-ICU patients. The only study describing the outcome of IDUs with RSIE needing ICU admission reported a mortality of 26% [2].

Some factors have been associated with a worse prognosis: acute respiratory failure requiring mechanical ventilation, shock, Simplified Acute Physiology Score (SAPS II) $\geq$ 20, and Sequential Organ Failure Assessment (SOFA) $\geq$ 3 [2, 5].

Other elements that play an essential role at the 30-day survival are age <45 years, Charlson score < 3, endocarditis diagnosed before ICU admission, aminoglycoside use, the presence of septic pulmonary embolism, and a single surgical indication for patients needing a surgical procedure [2].

Reasons for admission to the ICU were a congestive cardiac failure (64%), septic shock (21%), neurological deterioration (15%), and cardiopulmonary resuscitation (9%). Younger patients have a better prognosis because they usually present a minimal dysfunction of the right-sided valve, low risk of pulmonary embolism, and reasonable response to appropriate antibiotic therapy [2].

Opposite to the last IE guidelines, which no longer recommend the aminoglycosides in the treatment of native valve staphylococcal endocarditis, Georges et al. found a better survival in their patients treated with a combination of penicillins or vancomycin with gentamicin [2].

7. Risk factors

It is imperative to describe this pathology in the people with susceptible risk factors (**Table 2**).

7.1 RSIE in people with intravenous drug addiction (IVDA)

The majority of cases of RSIE reports in the literature are in drug abusers. This kind of populations of RSIE represents the 32–86% of all IE [2, 3].

There are multiple explanations about the preference of infection in the right side of the heart at this group of the population, being the leading causes of the poor hygiene with unsafe injection practices and the affected immunology well-being. The higher bacterial load and the variety of effects of injected substances over the endocardium also play an essential role in the physiopathology of the infection [7].

Intravenous drugs abuser´s	Indwelling catheters	Intracardiac devices	Congenital heart diseases
32-86% cases of RSIE	HD patients in risk of bacteremia and IE	Worse prognosis and mortality (11-36%)	IE more often is adults than pediatrics
Reinfection 28%, reoperation 20%	Incidence of 8% of all IE	Removal of the infected device is mandatory	VSD is the main anomaly in RSIE
HIV association doesn´t increase mortality	AVF diminish risk of IE		Stretococci and Staphylococci are the most frequent bacterias
Survival is equal in comparison with not drug abusers	Noncuffed catheters increase risk of IE		

AVF: arteriovenous fistula, HD: hemodialytic, HIV: human immunodeficiency virus, IE: infective endocarditis, RSIE: right-sided infected endocarditis, VSD: ventricular septal defect.

Table 2.
Characteristics of principal risk factors in the right-sided infective endocarditis.

The incidence of reinfections and reoperations is about 28 and 20%, respectively; however, the survival described in some papers is almost equal between drug abusers and not drug abusers, in which results are very striking [7].

Sometimes IVDA also presents human immunodeficiency virus (HIV) which can aggravate the predisposition to IE if this disease is not well-controlled. The death rates in this subgroup of patients are about 5–10% [1]. The HIV affects both humoral and cellular immunities which provoked a predisposition for recurrent episodes of bacteremia that cause valve damage, fibrin deposition, thrombus formation, and adherence by bacteria in the endocardium; it is common to find abscess developments and large vegetations, which are indications for early surgical treatment [18].

The choice of empiric antimicrobial therapy depends on the suspected microorganism and type of drug and solvent used by the addict and the location of infection.

As previously was described, the empirical antimicrobial therapy must cover *S. aureus*; the combination of penicillinase-resistant penicillins or vancomycin or daptomycin with gentamicin is recommended [5].

The 2015 ESC IE guidelines recommend an antipseudomonal therapy in patients with pentazocine addiction if IE is suspected; nevertheless, there are few and relatively old studies about this issue [5, 19, 20].

If an IVDA uses brown heroin dissolved in lemon juice, *Candida* spp. (not *Candida albicans*) should be considered and antifungal treatment added [5].

7.2 RSIE in people with no IVDA

Although the majority of IE at the right side of the heart is fairly reported in IVDA, there is an increasing incidence in another type of patients, mainly highlighting the people with indwelling catheters and cardiac devices. The 5–10% of RSIE occur in nonaddicted patients [3].

7.2.1 Indwelling catheters

It is estimated that more than 3 million people worldwide require dialysis for end-stage renal disease, and this number is expected to rise sharply because of the aging of the population and an increasing prevalence of diabetes and cardiovascular comorbidities paralleled by a decline in cardiovascular mortality, particularly in very elderly patients (>80 years). For instance, in the United States, this augmentation is about 3.2% per year [21, 22].

Hemodialysis patients are at increased risk for bacteremia, including an estimated 37,000 central line-associated bloodstream infections related to outpatient hemodialysis in the United States in 2008. The elevated incidence of bacteremia increases the risk for infective endocarditis [22, 23].

The average duration on HD before the diagnosis of IE was 30 months (range, 4–66 months). IE is one of the most important causes of increased mortality and morbidity among hemodialysis patients [24].

The *European Heart Journal* states that more than two-thirds of patients undergoing hemodialysis suffer from some infection and that one-third of these patients experience IE [24].

IE occurs 18 times more frequently in chronic HD patients than in the general population [25, 26].

The use of temporal or permanent central catheters, the constant puncture of arteriovenous fistulas, the long and frequent hospitalizations that some of these patients have to suffer during their disease, the various surgical procedures related with the creation of fistulas, and the underlying alteration of their defenses become susceptible to this population to develop IE.

The IE in HD patients is calculated about at 8% of all observed IE cases regarding the largest international cohort collected to date [27].

The incidence of IE usually increases with the time after the initiation of hemodialysis; however, some studies found a rise of this incidence in the first 5 months after the initiation of hemodialysis [26, 28]. This contradictory results can be probably due to the aseptic technique during the manipulation of the catheter and arteriovenous fistulas of these patients.

Patients in HD also present an increase in the incidence of endocarditis after aortic valve replacement surgery, affecting at the same time the short-term and long-term survival [22].

Most of the studies show that central catheters are a risk factor for bacteremia and endocarditis [6, 7, 10]; nevertheless, Farrington et al. did not find an increase of endocarditis in patients with central catheters in comparison with patients with arteriovenous fistulas [22].

Besides, the rates of IE are more significant in patients with non-cuffed catheters than cuffed catheters; the vascular grafts have more incidence of IE than AV fistulas. Furthermore, peritoneal dialysis has then lesser rates of IE due to the lack of contact of the line with luminal vessels [29].

The morbidity and mortality are higher than the general population; in the 20% of hemodialysis-related IE, the tricuspid valve is the principal place affected at the right side of the heart.

The pathogenesis of IE in HD patient can be attributed to recurrent episodes of bacteremia, the immunological compromise of hemodialytic patients and heart valvular deterioration-calcification frequently founded in this patients.

It can sound logical that the majority of cases of IE in HD patients should happen on the right cavities, similar to what occurs in IVDA; however, the left-side heart (90%) is the more frequent infected place in HD patients, the mitral being the main valve affected. The affectation of the right cavities is roughly 10%. Nevertheless, some papers report an incidence of RSIE in HD patients of between 0 and 50% [30, 31].

Between the multiple explanations of pathogenesis RSIE in HD patients, the high turbulent flow throughout the valves can provoke a deterioration at these structures, becoming more susceptible to bacterial implantation. Nonetheless, the low pressures at the right cavities might not present the same effect in their valves. One possible cause can be the associated pulmonary hypertension that some patients express, due to multiple factors, such as an increased cardiac output (hypervolemic condition and arteriovenous fistula), an increased pulmonary vascular resistance (uremic endothelial dysfunction and pulmonary artery calcifications), and elevated pulmonary capillary wedge pressure caused by heart failure or mitral valve disease [17].

7.2.1.1 Prevention

Patients in HD have an increased risk of developing IE due to all the reasons described before, so to take some measurements sounds logical to diminish the incidence of bacteremia which can result in an IE.

In some hospitals, their politics have been changed regarding the hemodialysis procedure with the intention to ameliorate the arteriovenous life expectancy and decrease the local and systemic infections. For instance, Oun HA et al. have published a lowering in the bacteremia and IE at his hospital adopting new strategies, such as changing the lock solution to taurolidine, cleaning the puncture site with chlorhexidine 2%, and using the buttonhole technique instead of the rope ladder technique.

Nonetheless, it is important to mention that the buttonhole technique had a modest but not significative rising of bacteremia following the move to buttonhole [26].

The arteriovenous fistula (AVF) must always be the best option to perform HD due to their low rates of bacteremia and IE, so, it is imperative to develop an adequate surgical technique and improve the care of the fistula. Whenever it is possible, the fistula must be carried out at the distal part of the arms, trying to preserve the proximal areas to future AVF if the distal fistula fails at some point. If the HD needs a temporary or permanent catheter, the cuffed ones always are preferable to non-cuffed catheters, because the former cause fewer rates of IE [29].

The patient and healthcare personnel must be informed and trained regarding the proper care of the AVF and catheters to lower the probability of bacteremia and IE. The cleaning of the surgical area is paramount as well as the correct AVF puncture.

7.2.2 Intracardiac devices (ICD)

Nowadays ICD are widely used worldwide; their implementation in the cardiology area has improved the quality of life of many people and increased the survival; nonetheless, they have side defects, the endocarditis being one of the most severe complications.

The IE on a cardiac device is increased in the last 10 years in the first-world countries, even becoming the most common cause of IE in some regions. This phenomenon is caused mainly by the rise in the longevity in these countries which results in a growing number of intracardiac devices implanted (pacemakers, cardiac defibrillator, cardiac resynchronizer, or ventricle assist device) [32].

This IE is associated with a worse prognosis and high mortality (11–36%) [32–34]. The pacemaker generator or lead change is the higher factor of risk for IE on the cardiac device. The tricuspid valve is the most common site of RSIE associated with this kind of devices [7, 35].

The removal of the infected device is mandatory in the treatment of intracardiac device infective endocarditis (ICDIE) because it decreases the hospital mortality [32]. Patients with device-related infection and intracardiac vegetations higher or equal at 1 cm have historically undergone surgery for device removal due to the potential risk for septic embolization [34].

7.2.3 Congenital heart disease (CHD)

The risk of IE in patients with adult congenital heart disease (ACHD) is substantially higher (15–140 times) than in the general population. The RSIE in CHD is more often in adults than pediatric patients [5, 36].

The ventricular septal defect (VSD) is the most frequent anomaly in right-sided IE with an incidence of 0.2–2% of all IE [37].

The risk of IE can occur either in repaired or not repaired VSD, with a higher increase in the last one [38].

A recent paper from Tutarel et al. found an incidence of 15.9% of IE in patients with VSD; the 50% of these cases were associated with infections of either the tricuspid valve or the right ventricular outflow tract [36].

The 2015 ESC IE guidelines describe that the distribution of causative organisms does not differ from the pattern found in acquired heart disease, with streptococci and staphylococci being the most common strains. Another study found the streptococci responsible for 50% of congenital heart disease infective endocarditis (CHDIE) and the staphylococci with a 31% incidence [5, 36].

The pulmonary valve is affected in almost 32% of patients from which over an 84% are prosthetic and near 16% native valve [36].

8. Locations

Unlike the left-sided IE mainly occurring on the aorta or mitral valve, right-sided IE could involve the tricuspid valve (82%), pulmonary valve, eustachian valve, interventricular septum, right ventricular free wall, or CS [4, 9].

8.1 Tricuspid valve (TV)

The vast majority of RSIE cases involve the TV (approximately 90%). The high risk of vegetations on the TV is septic PE resulting in various pulmonary complications such as pneumonia and pulmonary abscess.

Uncomplicated tricuspid valve endocarditis can be successfully treated medically in 80% of patients and in the remaining 20% with very large vegetations and expectably poor antibiotic penetration [6].

The infection of the native tricuspid valve in nonaddicted adults occurs in younger patients (under 50 years). In the majority of cases (70%), there are underlying medical conditions such as alcoholism, abortion, colon disease, immunodeficiency, permanent catheters, septic processes in the oral cavity, skin, or genitals, etc. The 25% of cases require valve replacement or surgery [3] (**Figure 2**).

8.2 Pulmonary valve (PV)

RSIE in PV happens in less than 10% of the patients [7]. Most of the cases of pulmonary valve infective endocarditis (PVIE) are provoked by prosthetic material present at this place due to previous surgeries or interventional procedures focused on figuring a congenital disease out.

Bovine jugular grafts are associated with a significantly higher risk of late endocarditis compared with homografts [39].

However, Robichaud et al. did not find an increased risk of PVIE regarding the type of valve, including bovine jugular vein grafts [40].

The rate of IE in transcatheter pulmonary valve implantation is higher than surgical homograft implantation [41].

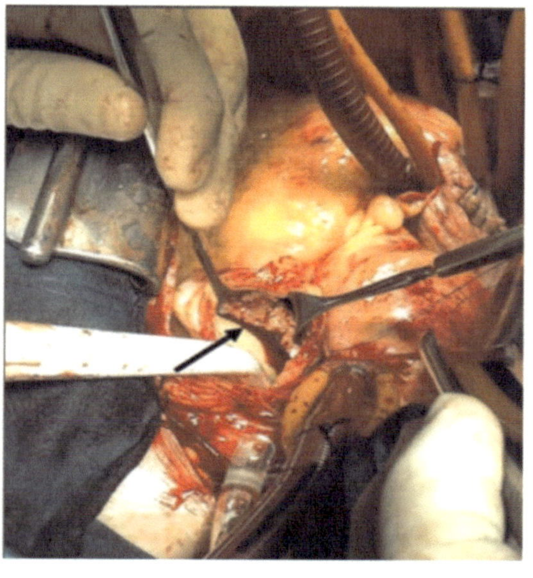

Figure 2.
Pulmonary native endocarditis: a giant mass anchored to the posterior leaflet of pulmonary valve [42].

8.3 Other sites

Uniquely few case reports have been published about RSIE in other locations different to tricuspid and pulmonary valves.

8.3.1 Eustachian valve

Reports of eustachian valve infective endocarditis (EVIE) are approximately 29 cases [43]. An incidence of 3.3% in patients with right-sided endocarditis has been reported [44].

Eustachian valve is a rudimentary structure in adults and, during fetal life, directs oxygenated blood from the inferior vena cava through the foramen ovale and into the left atrium [43, 45].

IVDA is the main high-risk population to develop an EVIE (over 50% of cases). *Staphylococcus aureus* is the most common bacteria implicated in this process [43]. TOE is necessary to identify the vegetation at eustachian valve because this structure is not accessible with TTE [45].

8.3.2 Coronary sinus

There are only eight reported cases of IE in the coronary sinus (CS). The clinical manifestations, the complementary test, the responsible bacteria, and antibiotic treatment are very similar to the other RSIE locations. The CSIE has some features; the CS is always dilated and generally the only affected valve; the vegetation is usually mobile and has a tubule shape with a length of >10 mm [9, 46].

9. Conclusions

RSIE is a pathology scarcely studied because there are few articles released about it. One of the significant reasons about the RSIE little information is the low incidence of this disease; nevertheless, the rates of frequency of this infection are rising nowadays due to the steady increase of HD patients and implanted ICD.

- RSIE clinic criteria are necessary to establish to help in the diagnosis of the disease, such as modified Duke criteria.

- Healthcare personnel must be aware of this illness, keeping their suspicion in high-risk patients and performing the proper complementary test to confirm or discard this infection.

- Hospital policies should be continuously updated to diminish the incidence of RSIE, an adequate epidemiologic analysis about RSIE cases, the population in potential risk to acquire the infection, and the most frequent bugs implicated in this one.

Conflict of interest

None.

DOI: http://dx.doi.org/10.5772/intechopen.85019

Nomenclature

ACHD	adult congenital heart disease
AVF	arteriovenous fistula
CHD	congenital heart disease
CHDIE	congenital heart disease infective endocarditis
CS	coronary sinus
CT	computed tomography
EVIE	eustachian valve infective endocarditis
HD	hemodialytic
HIV	human immunodeficiency virus
ICD	intracardiac devices
ICU	intensive care unit
IE	infective endocarditis
IIAs	infectious intracranial aneurysms
IVDA	intravenous drugs addiction
LSIE	left-side infective endocarditis
MRSA	methicillin-resistant *Staphylococcus aureus*
MR	magnetic resonance
PET	positron-emission tomography
PE	pulmonary embolism
PVIE	prosthetic valve infective endocarditis
PV	pulmonary valve
RSIE	right-side infective endocarditis
SAPS	Simplified Acute Physiology Score
SOFA	sequential organ failure assessment
TTE	transthoracic echocardiography
TOE	transesophageal echocardiography
TV	tricuspid valve
VSD	ventricle septal defect

Author details

Adrian Fernando Narvaez Muñoz[1*] and Daniela Albina Ibarra Vargas[2]

1 Department of Cardiovascular Surgery, Hospital de Especialidades Dr. Abel Gilbert Pontón, Guayaquil Clinic, Guayaquil, Ecuador

2 Department of Cardiology, Hospital de Especialidades Dr. Abel Gilbert Pontón, Guayaquil, Ecuador

*Address all correspondence to: adrianfnm@hotmail.com

References

[1] Horimoto K, Kubo T, Matsusaka H, Baba H, Umesue M. Right-sided infective endocarditis with a ruptured sinus of Valsalva and multiple septic pulmonary emboli in a patient with atopic dermatitis. Internal Medicine. 2015;**54**(7):797-800

[2] Georges H, Leroy O, Airapetian N, Lamblin N, Zogheib E, Devos P, et al. Outcome and prognostic factors of patients with right-sided infective endocarditis requiring intensive care unit admission. BMC Infectious Diseases. 2018;**18**(1):85

[3] Varona J, Guerra J. Tricuspid valve endocarditis in a nonaddicted patient without predisposing myocardiopathy. Revista Española de Cardiología. 2004; **57**:993-996

[4] Revilla A, López J, Villacorta E, Gómez I, Sevilla T, del Pozo MA, et al. Endocarditis derecha aislada en pacientes no adictos a drogas por vía parenteral. Revista Española de Cardiología. 2008;**61**(12):1253-1259

[5] Habib G, Lancellotti P, Antunes MJ, Bongiorni MG, Casalta JP, Del Zott F. 2015 ESC Guidelines for the management of infective endocarditis: The task force for the management of infective endocarditis of the European Society of Cardiology (ESC) Endorsed by: European Association for Cardio-Thoracic Surgery (EACTS), the European Association of Nuclear Medicine (EANM). European Heart Journal. 2015;**36**(44):3075-3128

[6] Weymann A, Schmack B, Rosendal C, Rauch H, Karck M, Tochtermann U, et al. Tricuspid valve endocarditis with septic pulmonary emboli in a drug addict. British Heart Journal. 1990; **63**(6):368-369

[7] Hussain ST, Witten J, Shrestha NK, Blackstone EH, Pettersson GB. Tricuspid valve endocarditis. The Annals of Cardiothoracic Surgery. 2017; **6**(3):255-261

[8] Póvoa P, Salluh JI. Biomarker-guided antibiotic therapy in adult critically ill patients: A critical review. Annals of Intensive Care. 2012;**2**(1):32

[9] Song G, Zhang J, Zhang X, Yang H, Huang W, Du M, et al. Right-sided infective endocarditis with coronary sinus vegetation. BMC Cardiovascular Disorders. 2018;**18**(1):111

[10] Hryniewiecki T, Zatorska K, Abramczuk E, Zakrzewski D, Szymański P, Kuśmierczyk M, et al. The usefulness of cardiac CT in the diagnosis of perivalvular complications in patients with infective endocarditis. European Radiology. 2019. DOI: 10.1007/s00330-018-5965-2

[11] Migdady I, Rice CJ, Hassett C, Zhang LQ, Wisco D, Uchino K, et al. MRI presentation of infectious intracranial aneurysms in infective endocarditis. Neurocritical Care. 2018. DOI: 10.1007/s12028-018-0654-1

[12] Álvarez Velasco R, Salvat Dávila C, Vigil Díaz C. Usefulness of PET scan in the diagnosis of infective endocarditis. Medicina Clínica (Barcelona). 2018. DOI: 10.1016/j.medcli.2018.07.017

[13] Diemberger I, Bonfiglioli R, Martignani C, Graziosi M, Biffi M, Lorenzetti S, et al. Contribution of PET imaging to mortality risk stratification in candidates to lead extraction for pacemaker or defibrillator infection: A prospective single center study. European Journal of Nuclear Medicine and Molecular Imaging. 2019;**46**(1): 194-205

[14] Carozza A, Renzulli A, De Feo M, Ismeno G, Della Corte A, Dialetto G, et al. Tricuspid repair for infective

endocarditis: Clinical and echocardiographic results. Annals of Thoracic and Cardiovascular Surgery. 2012;**18**(5):481-484

[15] Durden RE, Turek JW, Reinking BE, Bansal M. Acquired ventricular septal defect due to infective endocarditis. Annals of Pediatric Cardiology. 2018; **11**(1):100-102

[16] Arbulu A, Holmes RJ, Asfaw I. Tricuspid valvulectomy without replacement. Twenty years' experience. The Journal of Thoracic and Cardiovascular Surgery. 1991;**102**(6): 917-922

[17] Zea-Vera R, Sanchez M, Castañeda E, Soto-Arquiñigo L. Surgical management of multiple valve endocarditis associated with dialysis catheter. Case Reports in Infectious Diseases. 2016;**2016**:4072056

[18] Cicalini S, Forcina G, De Rosa FG. Infective endocarditis in patients with human immunodeficiency virus infection. Journal of Infection. 2001;**42**: 267-271

[19] Shekar R, Rice TW, Zierdt CH, Kallick CA. Outbreak of endocarditis caused by *Pseudomonas aeruginosa* serotype O11 among pentazocine and tripelennamine abusers in Chicago. The Journal of Infectious Diseases. 1985; **151**(2):203-208

[20] Wieland M, Lederman MM, Kline-King C, Keys TF, Lerner PI, Bass SN, et al. Left-sided endocarditis due to *Pseudomonas aeruginosa*. A report of 10 cases and review of the literature. Medicine (Baltimore). 1986;**65**(3): 180-189

[21] Viecelli AK, Lok CE. Hemodialysis vascular access in the elderly-getting it right. Kidney International. 2019;**95**(1): 38-49

[22] Farrington DK, Kilgo PD, Thourani VH, Jacob JT, Steinberg JP. High risk of prosthetic valve endocarditis and death after valve replacement operations in dialysis patients. The Annals of Thoracic Surgery. 2016;**101**(6):2217-2223

[23] Ishida K, Brown MG, Weiner M, Kobrin S, Kasner SE, Messé SR. Endocarditis is a common stroke mechanism in hemodialysis patients. Stroke. 2014;**45**:1164-1166

[24] Habib Khan Y, Sarriff A, Hayat Khan A, Azreen Syazril A, Mallhi TH. Infective endocarditis and chronic kidney disease: How to deal with complications. The Malaysian Journal of Medical Sciences. 2015;**22**(4):73-75

[25] Omoto T, Aoki A, Maruta K, Masuda T. Surgical outcome in hemodialysis patients with active-phase infective endocarditis. Annals of Thoracic and Cardiovascular Surgery. 2016;**22**(3):181-185

[26] Oun HA, Price AJ, Traynor JP. Infective endocarditis in patients on haemodialysis–Possible strategies for prevention. Scottish Medical Journal. 2016;**61**(2):97-102

[27] Murdoch DR, Corey GR, Hoen B, International collaboration on endocarditis-prospective (ICE-PCS) Investigators, et al. Clinical presentation, etiology and outcome of infective endocarditis in the 21st century: The International Collaboration on endocarditis-prospective cohort study. Archives of Internal Medicine. 2009;**169**(5):463-473

[28] Chaudry MS, Carlson N, Gislason GH, Kamper AL, Rix M, Fowler VG Jr, et al. Risk of infective endocarditis in patients with end stage renal disease. Clinical Journal of the American Society of Nephrology. 2017;**12**(11):1814-1822

[29] Bentata Y. Physiopathological approach to infective endocarditis in chronic hemodialysis patients: Left heart

versus right heart involvement. Renal Failure. 2017;**39**(1):432-439

[30] Krcmery V, Kisac P. Bacterial endocarditis in haemodialysis patients. Is frequent heparinisation protecting embolisation? European Journal of Clinical Microbiology & Infectious Diseases. 2011;**30**:1627-1628

[31] Bentata Y, Haddiya I, Ismailli N, et al. Infective endocarditis in chronic hemodialysis: A transition from left heart to right heart? Saudi Journal of Kidney Diseases and Transplantation. 2016;**27**:1200-1206

[32] Ortiz-Bautista C, López J, García-Granja PE, Vilacosta I, Sevilla T, Sarriá C, et al. Endocarditis infecciosa derecha en portadores de dispositivos cardiacos: Perfil clínico y pronóstico. Medicina Clínica. 2017;**149**:477-482. DOI: 10.1016/j.medcli.2017.03.055

[33] Chu VH. Clinical characteristics and outcome of infective endocarditis involving implantable cardiac devices. Journal of the American Medical Association. 2012;**307**:1727. DOI: 10.1001/jama.2012.497

[34] Grammes JA, Schulze CM, Al-Bataineh M, Yesenosky GA, Saari CS, Vrabel MJ, et al. Percutaneous pacemaker and implantable cardioverter-defibrillator lead extraction in 100 patients with intracardiac vegetations defined by transesophageal echocardiogram. Journal of the American College of Cardiology. 2010;**55**:886-894. DOI: 10.1016/j.jacc.2009.11.03

[35] Xu Z, Shi Q, Mei J, Tan Y. Bioprosthetic tricuspid valve replacement for tricuspid valve endocarditis secondary to infected endocardial pacemaker leads. Journal of Cardiac Surgery. 2017;**32**:5-8. DOI: 10.1111/jocs.12878

[36] Tutarel O, Alonso-Gonzalez R, Montanaro C, Schiff R, Uribarri A, Kempny A, et al. Infective endocarditis in adults with congenital heart disease remains a lethal disease. Heart. 2018; **104**(2):161-165

[37] Lee M-R, Chang S-A, Choi S-H, Lee G-Y, Kim E-K, Peck K-R, et al. Clinical features of right-sided infective endocarditis occurring in non-drug users. Journal of Korean Medical Science. 2014;**29**:776-781

[38] Lee PT, Uy FM, Foo JS, Tan JL. Increased incidence of infective endocarditis in patients with ventricular septal defect. Congenital Heart Disease. 2018;**13**(6):1005-1011

[39] Mery CM, Guzman-Pruneda FA, De Leon LE, Zhang W, Terwelp MD, Bocchini CE, et al. Risk factors for development of endocarditis and reintervention in patients undergoing right ventricle to pulmonary artery valved conduit placement. The Journal of Thoracic and Cardiovascular Surgery. 2016;**151**:432-439. 441.e1-2

[40] Robichaud B, Hill G, Cohen S, Woods R, Earing M, Frommelt P, et al. Bioprosthetic pulmonary valve endocarditis: Incidence, risk factors, and clinical outcomes. Congenital Heart Disease. 2018;**13**(5):734-739

[41] Van Dijck I, Budts W, Cools B, Eyskens B, Boshoff DE, Heying R, et al. Infective endocarditis of a transcatheter pulmonary valve in comparison with surgical implants. Heart. 2015;**101**: 788-793

[42] Narvaez A, Granda A, Sierra J, Adrio B, Reija L. Aortic and pulmonary endocarditis with hemorrhagic stroke complication: Which is the ideal surgical time? Cirugia Cardiovascular. 2016;**23**: 255-258

[43] Kottam A, Kaur R, Bhandare D, Zmily H, Bheemreddy S, Brar H, et al. Actinomycotic endocarditis of the eustachian valve: A rare case and a review of the literature. Texas Heart Institute Journal. 2015;**42**(1):44-49. DOI: 10.14503/THIJ-13-3517

[44] San Román JA, Vilacosta I, Sarriá C, Garcimartín I, Rollán MJ, Fernández-Avilés F. Eustachian valve endocarditis: Is it worth searching for? American Heart Journal. 2001;**142**(6):1037-1040

[45] Mordi I, Tzemos N. Think twice, look twice: Eustachian valve endocarditis due to *Escherichia coli*. Journal of Cardiology Cases. 2012;7(2): e51-e52. DOI: 10.1016/j.jccase. 2012.10.003

[46] Machado MN, Nakazone MA, Takakura IT, Silva CM, Maia LN. Spontaneous bacterial pericarditis and coronary sinus endocarditis caused by oxacillin-susceptible *Staphylococcus aureus*. Case Reports in Medicine. 2010; **2010**:984562. DOI: 10.1155/2010/984562

Chapter 4

Infective Endocarditis in Intravenous Drug Users: Surgical Treatment

Moldovan Horatiu, Adrian Molnar, Victor Costache and Ecaterina Bontas

Abstract

Intravenous drug use is associated with infective endocarditis. Besides, it does appear that left-sided infective endocarditis is a feature of general population, whereas right-sided infective endocarditis is common in intravenous drug users. The most common etiology of right-sided infective endocarditis in intravenous drug users is *Staphylococcus aureus* in about 75% followed by streptococci, Gram-negative bacilli and fungi. In case of intravenous drug users with infective endocarditis, optimal treatment strategies lack a general consensus. Additionally, the best indication and timing of surgery are debatable. To overcome these problems, the early and complete surgical debridement of infected tissue together with microbial therapy assures a good prognosis in the long term.

Keywords: endocarditis, drug-associated endocarditis, intravenous drug abuser endocarditis, intravenous drug users, right heart endocarditis

1. Introduction

Infective endocarditis (IE) is a rare infectious disease with elevated morbidity and mortality [1]. Intravenous drug use is associated with infective endocarditis (IE) [2]. To the best of our knowledge, IE accounts for 2–5% per year among the intravenous drug users (IDUs) [3–6]. Approximately 41% of IDUs with bacteremia will develop IE [7]. Conversely, it is widely agreed that intravenous drug users (IDUs) diagnosed with IE are mainly white young males [8–12].

Right-sided infective endocarditis has been mainly defined among IDUs [13–15]. Generally, right-sided IE comprises 5–10% of cases with IE [16–18]. It does appear that left-sided IE is a feature of general population, whereas right-sided IE is common in IDUs [19–21]. To further characterize, IDUs may present in 86% cases right-sided IE, whereas 14% have left-sided IE with or without right-sided IE [21]. However, some older data outlines that the IDUs group may present equal incidence of left-sided and right-sided IE [22].

Common ***predisposing factors*** for right-sided IE are the intravenous drug users (IDUs), catheter-related infections, pacemaker or defibrillators wires, intracardiac devices (catheters for hemodialysis; tricuspid prosthetic valve), right heart catheterization, congenital heart defects, sepsis, and alcoholism [13–15, 23]. In case of the right-sided IE, tricuspid valve is affected in 90% cases [21], whereas pulmonic valve represents about 10% from right-sided IE cases [3, 18, 24]. Up to now, isolated right-sided IE involving the pulmonary valve, the eustachian valve, interventricular septum, or right ventricular free wall have been described [17, 21, 25].

2. Microbiology

According to current evidence, IE among IDUs presents a large spectrum of microbial pathogens (**Table 1**) [26–31].

Pathogens as *Pseudomonas aeruginosa*, other gram-negative microorganisms, fungi, enterococci, streptococci, and polymicrobial infections occur less frequently [16]. Importantly, other pathogens noted in IDUs are oral bacteria such as *Prevotella intermedia*, *Haemophilus parainfluenzae*, *S. constellatus*, and *E. corrodens* [32–36].

The most common etiology of right-sided IE in IDUs is *Staphylococcus aureus (S. aureus)* in about 75% [1, 4, 6, 37–39] followed by streptococci, Gram-negative bacilli, and fungi [40]. In fact, published data supports the involvement of *S. aureus* among IDUs in 40–74% cases of IE [38, 41, 42]. *S. aureus* is the most common cause of tricuspid valve endocarditis regardless of associated risk factors in IDUs [1, 4, 16, 18, 43].

The incidence of negative blood cultures is reported as 2.5–31% and is associated with delayed diagnosis and treatment [44], with large vegetations [45], and with highest morbidity and mortality [16, 45, 46].

Regarding HIV, a prevalence of HIV as high as 60% among IDUs has been reported by centers from Europe and the USA [11, 40]. HIV is more common among IDUs with right-sided IE than left-sided IE [47].

Polymicrobial endocarditis is characteristically for IDUs [48] and may involve microorganisms such as *Bartonella* spp., *Candida* spp., or *Tropheryma whipplei* [49]. The presence of *E. corrodens* should aware the likelihood of polymicrobial IE with embolic complications and relapses. In fact, there is a synergism between streptococci and *E. corrodens* [50–52].

- *Staphylococcus aureus* and coagulase-negative staphylococci,
- group A streptococci,
- *P. aeruginosa*,
- HACEK organisms (*Haemophilus aphrophilus*, *Actinobacillus actinomycetemcomitans*, *Cardiobacterium hominis*, *Eikenella corrodens*, and *Kingella kingae*),
- Tetanus (*Clostridium tetani*),
- Anthrax (*Bacillus anthracis*),
- wound botulism (*Clostridium botulinum*),
- tuberculosis,
- diphtheria (*Corynebacterium diphtheriae*),
- viruses (HIV, HBV with HDV, HCV, and HTLV),
- fungal infections (*Candida* spp. and *Aspergillus* spp.),
- parasitic infections (malaria and leishmaniasis)

Table 1.
Spectrum of microbial pathogens may constitute comorbidity in IDUs [26–31].

3. Diagnosis

History and classic Oslerian manifestations (persistent bacteremia or fungemia, active valvulitis, immunological vascular phenomena, and peripheral emboli) help with a straightforward diagnosis in IE [1]. Typical clinical manifestations of IE comprise fever, positive blood cultures, and valvular vegetations on echocardiography [53]. IE should be suspected in the presence of fever and embolic phenomena [16]. Persistent fever and bacteremia are common manifestations of tricuspid valve IE [16].

Clinical manifestations are usually limited in the early IE of IDUs, right-sided endocarditis and *S. aureus* [1]. Right-sided IE mainly present fever, cough, hemoptysis, dyspnea caused by pulmonary emboli, anemia, and no systemic emboli [23]. Characteristically, right-sided IE does not develop immunological vascular phenomena (splinter hemorrhages, Roth spots, and glomerulonephritis) and the peripheral emboli [1]. Right-sided IE can be associated with septic pulmonary emboli [1]. In fact, pulmonary embolism is often present in right-sided IE and pacemaker wires IE [16].

Usually, the association of clinical findings, positive blood cultures, and positive echocardiography set up the diagnosis [23]. However, these typical clinical manifestations of IE are often absent among IDUs, especially in those infected with *S. aureus* and HACEK (*Haemophilus species*, *Actinobacillus actinomycetemcomitans*, *Cardiobacterium hominis*, *Eikenella corrodens*, *Kingella kingae*) [54]. Common complications of right-sided IE are valvular regurgitations, cardiac abscess, and septic pulmonary emboli [55].

Relapse and reinfection are two types of recurrence [16]. Basically, recurrence within 6 months of same IE produced by same microorganisms is termed ***relapse*** [55]. Reinfection or recurrent IE refers to the ***recurrence*** of same IE with same microorganisms after 6 months from initial episode [53]. Recurrent IE has higher frequency in IDUs with increased valve replacement [16] with a reported incidence as 41% [56].

The landmark lesion of IE is the ***vegetation*** (**Figure 1**) [57]. In this context, IDUs population with vegetations >20 mm may present higher embolic risk [58] and higher mortality as well [25, 58, 59].

The cornerstone of imaging diagnosing for infective endocarditis is echocardiography [16]. Transthoracic echocardiography (TTE) and/or transesophageal echocardiography (TOE) are vital in the diagnosis of any IE [16]. TTE is the first line recommendation either for native valve endocarditis or for prosthetic valve endocarditis. In case of suspected native valve endocarditis, TTE has a sensitivity of 50–90% and a specificity of 90% [60]. For IE with vegetation, TTE has a moderate sensitivity (75%) and high specificity (>90%) [61]. For suspected prosthetic valve endocarditis, TTE has a reduced sensitivity of 40–70%. However, TTE comes up with significant information regarding ventricular size and function, and "hemodynamic severity of valve lesions" [60]. Major criteria in the diagnosis of IE are represented by three echocardiographic features: vegetation, abscess or pseudoaneurysm, and prosthetic valve with new dehiscence [16]. Moreover, TTE provides useful information in the diagnosis of anterior prosthetic aortic valve abscesses, which are difficult to be seen on TEE [60].

TOE is recommended when TTE is nondiagnostic or positive, suspected complications, or in presence of intracardiac device leads [60]. In case of native valve endocarditis, TOE has a sensitivity of 90–100% and a specificity of 90% for revealing vegetations. As such, TOE is highly superior to TOE regarding the detection

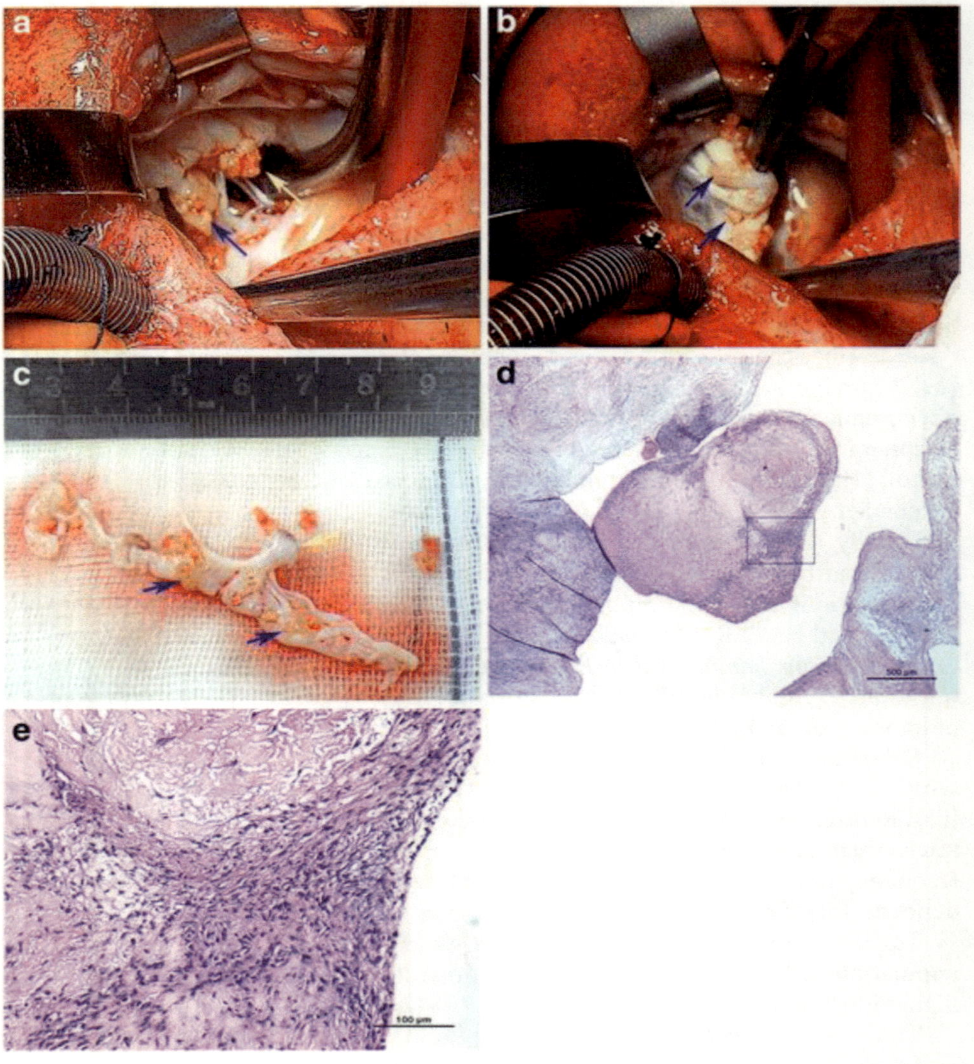

Figure 1.
Macroscopy and microscopy of the involved tricuspid valve and vegetation. (a) Yellow arrowhead: the large vegetation, blue arrowhead: rupture main chordae tendineae. (b) Blue arrowheads: multiple verrucous nodular vegetation on the atrial surface of leaflet. (c) Resected tricuspid valve. Blue arrowheads: multiple small vegetations, yellow arrowhead: rupture main chordae tendineae. (d) Microscopy of the vegetation adhered to the leaflet, magnification 4×, hematoxylin and Eosin stain. (e) Enlarged square area in (e) showing inflammatory cell infiltration and fibrin-platelet thrombi, magnification 20×, hematoxylin and Eosin stain. NOTE: every figure specifies this sentence beginning: From Bai et al. [57]. It is an open access article distributed under the terms of the Creative Commons Attribution License (http://creativecommons.org/licenses/by/4.0), which permits unrestricted use, distribution, and reproduction in any medium, provided the original work is properly credited.

of abscesses, perforations, and fistulae [60]. TOE has higher sensibility in the detection of pulmonary vegetations [62]. When clinical manifestations sustain IE with negative or unclear TTE, TOE has high sensitivity (>90%) and may reveal: (1) vegetations; (2) paravalvular or intracardiac abscess, (3) new valvular regurgitations, and (4) prosthetic valve dehiscence (**Figure 2**) [57, 63, 64].

Currently, 3D TOE provides useful information about the morphology and size of vegetation, evaluation of perivalvular extension, dehiscence of prosthetic valve, and valve perforation [65].

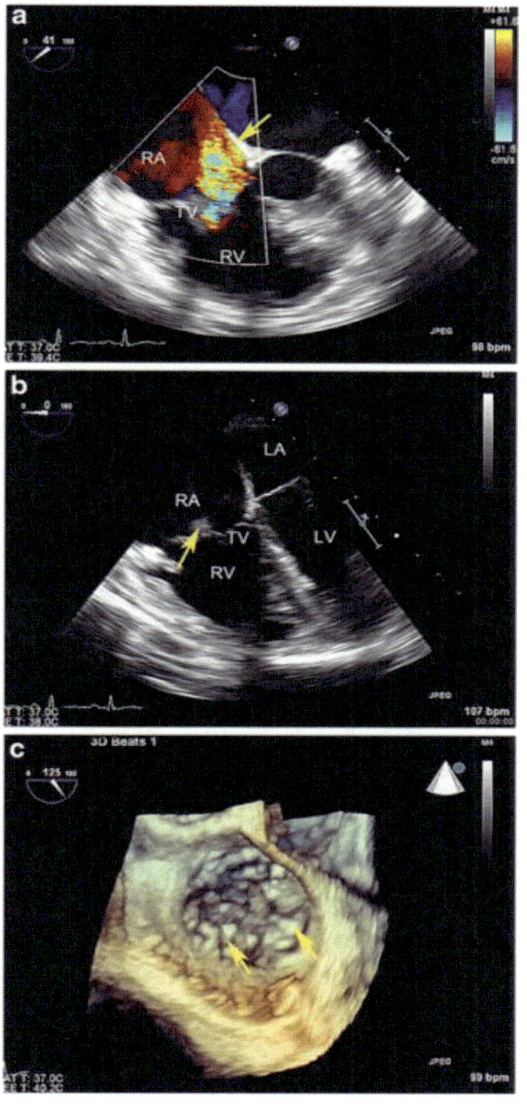

Figure 2.
Transesophageal echocardiography images of the patient before surgery. (a) Tricuspid regurgitation, Yellow arrowhead: wide and reversed blood flow signals at TV site. (b) A large vegetation formation. Yellow arrowhead: a large vegetation adheres to anterior leaflet of TV. (c) Suspicious multiple vegetations on 3D echo image. Yellow arrowheads: multiple verrucous abnormal nodular projections on the leaflet surface. RA right atrium, RV right ventricle, LA left atrium, LV left ventricle, TV tricuspid valve. NOTE: every figure specifies this sentence beginning: From Bai et al. [57]. It is an open access article distributed under the terms of the Creative Commons Attribution License (http://creativecommons.org/licenses/by/4.0), which permits unrestricted use, distribution, and reproduction in any medium, provided the original work is properly credited.

Other imaging techniques such as magnetic resonance imaging (MRI), multislice computed tomography (MSCT), and 18F-fluorodeoxyglucose (FDG) positron emission tomography (PET)/computed tomography (CT) are also valuable for the diagnosis of IE [16]. MSCT, MRI, and cardiac CT can provide greater information when compared with TEE regarding either paravalvular anatomy or complications (e.g. mycotic aneurysms, paravalvular abscesses) with lesser prosthetic valve artifacts [60]. Currently, using CT imaging in the diagnosis of paravalvular lesions is a major criterion in the 2015 ESC guidelines on IE [16].

Modified Duke criteria (2000) for diagnostic classification are well-known [64] and reviewed by 2015 ESC Guidelines for the management of infective endocarditis [16]. Only that, these modified Duke criteria have poorer diagnostic precision in the early diagnosis of IE from IDUs, which present fewer typical clinical manifestations [16]. The addition of imagistic techniques cardiac/whole-body CT scan, cerebral MRI, ^{18}F-FDG PET/CT, and radiolabelled leucocyte SPECT/CT may increase accuracy of the modified Duke criteria in IDUs. To sum up, these modified Duke criteria are useful, but they do not substitute the decision of a multidisciplinary team or of the "Endocarditis Team" that is defined later [16].

4. Treatment

The initial treatment of IE is empirical in majority of cases [1]. Consistent with published data, the main effective treatment is medical therapy, whilst surgery is a choice in smaller cases [16]. So that, medical treatment in right-sided IE of IDUs is usually effective with good prognosis up to 80% cases [16, 23, 66].

S. aureus is the most frequent cause of IE in IDUs; as a result, medical treatment should cover this pathogen [16]. Short courses of antimicrobial therapy in right-sided IE with *S. aureus* in IDUs assure high cure rates (>85%) [1].

A short course (2 weeks) with oxacillin or cloxacillin is mainly sufficient [16]. Initial therapy comprises penicillinase-resistant penicillins, vancomycin, or daptomycin in combination with gentamicin [16]. Short course (2 weeks) with oxacillin or cloxacillin is mainly efficient for isolated tricuspid IE with good compliance to therapy, vegetation <20 mm, MSSA, without empyema or other metastatic sites of infection, without prosthetic valve or left-sided IE, without cardiac/extracardiac complications and without severe immunosuppression (<200CD4 cells/μL) with/without AIDS. Anti-pseudomonas agent should be added in pentazocine addict [59]. Antifungal therapy for Candida spp. is added when an IDU utilizes brown heroin combined with lemon juice [67].

A traditional approach for the treatment of right-sided IE is the regimen formed from gentamicin with nafcillin or oxacillin. Another approach of IDUs with right-sided *S. aureus* IE and no other complications (e.g. aortic or mitral valve involvement, extra pulmonary infections or meningitis, renal failure, MRSA infection) is the antimicrobial coverage with short-course (2 weeks) of beta-lactam plus aminoglycoside that may be greatly successful [1]. Current guidelines still suggest the use of gentamicin, but some available data suggest that it might be unnecessary [68].

Moreover, daptomycin monotherapy is approved for the therapy of *S. aureus* bacteremia or right-sided *S. aureus* IE [69]. If laboratory evaluation shows opiate withdrawal, 10–20 mg of long-acting methadone can be prescribed until the regular doses are established [70].

To sum up, it is problematic to treat IE in IDUs because of the frequent exposures to virulent microorganisms; poor compliance with treatment; illegal drug use or withdrawal manifestations during hospitalization; opioid maintenance therapy; and early self-discharge or long hospitalization [70, 71]. Regardless of correct antimicrobial therapy, IDUs develop *relapsing IE* [56, 72, 73].

5. Surgery

Surgery is not a contraindication for IDUs with IE [4]. However, surgery indications are complex and are based on the clinical manifestations, associated risk factors (e.g. age, microorganisms, size of vegetation, perivalvular infection, embolism, heart failure, and other associated comorbidities) and the expertise of surgery team [1]. A multidisciplinary team or the "Endocarditis team" with knowledge in cardiology, infectious diseases, microbiologists, imaging, neurologists, neurosurgeons, and cardiothoracic surgery should provide decisions regarding the indication and timing of surgery [1]. Cardiac surgery in IDUs with IE aims to remove infection with hemodynamics stabilization hemodynamic may be suggested for IDUs [74].

In terms of surgery, right-sided IE has better outcomes than left-sided IE [1]. General approach of IDUs with right-sided IE is medical therapy and to delay as much as possible the use of valve prostheses [1].

Surgical treatment indications for right-sided IE are following [1, 16, 28, 75]:

- TV vegetations >20 mm after recurrent septic pulmonary emboli with or without right heart failure;
- Severe tricuspid regurgitation with right heart failure unresponsive to medical therapy;
- IE with fungi or persistent bacteremia with virulent microorganisms for at least 7 days (e.g., *S. aureus*, *P. aeruginosa*) regardless of the antimicrobial therapy.

5.1 Timing of surgery

Only 5–16% of IDUs needs surgery [76–78]. However, if left-sided IE has clear indications for early surgery, and the indications for early surgery in right-sided IE are not established presently [79].

The strategy to delay surgery until the microbial therapy is accomplished and may decrease morbidity and mortality rates significantly. In keeping with published data, *early surgery* is a choice in case of IE with *Staphylococcus aureus* or fungal infection [1, 16, 80]. Early surgery of tricuspid valve IE is considered when associates (1) atrial septal defect; (2) prosthetic valve endocarditis; (3) infected pacing leads; (4) indwelling catheters; and (5) simultaneous left-sided IE [81, 82]. Additionally, development of bacteremia or pulmonary septic emboli also has early surgery.

5.2 Surgical techniques

The *principles of surgery* for tricuspid valve IE comprise debridement of infected tissue; excision of vegetations with valve conservation or valve repair; and removal of the TV with its replacement [16, 76, 81]. In case of *native pulmonary valve*, its preservation is usually recommended. If pulmonary replacement is mandatory, the utilization of a homograft or xenograft is favored.

Various techniques that are used in cardiac surgery for right-sided IE [71, 81, 82]:

- vegetectomy (excision of vegetations)
- valvulectomy (total removal of valve leaflets and chordate tendineae)
- valvectomy (valve excision)
- reconstruction of the cusps (e.g. bicuspidization or conversion to a bicuspid valve)
- pericardial patch augmentation
- Kay's or De Vega's annuloplasty

- annuloplasty ring implantation
- synthetic or expanded polytetrafluoroethylene (PTFE) neo-chords
- valve replacement (bioprosthetic, mechanical prostheses).

Importantly, first line of surgical techniques in IDUs is vegetectomy and valve repair [23].

Valve repair is mainly achieved with autologous pericardial patch, artificial chordae, and simple annuloplasty with sutures (Kay's or De Vega annuloplasty) [23]. Ruptured chordae may be restored with polytetrafluoroethylene neo-chordae [16].

In a single perforated valve leaflet (cusp) can be used either untreated or glutaraldehyde-treated autologous or bovine pericardial patch [16]. ***Pericardial patch reconstruction*** aims to avoid the use of any prosthetic materials [23]. Autologous pericardial patch repairs small defects by direct closure in case of one leaflet. It is also used in wide excision or debridement of one leaflet or two leaflets [23].

Bicuspidalization annuloplasty is done after total excision of the posterior leaflet of tricuspid valve. Importantly, septal leaflet excision of TV has high risk of postoperative atrio-ventricular block [23]. This technique is accomplished either by Kay's annuloplasty or De Vega annuloplasty. Both Kay's annuloplasty and De Vega annuloplasty are the first choices indication for valve repair mainly in IDUs [23]. After broad resection (>75%) of the anterior leaflet of TV, it is recommended using of prosthetic or pericardial annular ring [23].

Kay's annuloplasty is mainly done after the total resection of a leaflet, and it is accomplished by the placement of fixing sutures in the corresponding segment of annulus to create a bicuspid valve [23].

De Vega annuloplasty (**Figures 3** and **4**) is based on fixing of two semi-circular purse string sutures between the anteroseptal commissure to the posteroseptal commissure with tricuspid annular reduction [23, 83]. This leads to the coaptation of the residual two leaflets.

Valve replacement. Valve replacement is *required* in case of a large destroyed valve with increased pulmonary pressures and pulmonary vascular resistance [16, 76, 81]. It also requires the absence of drug addiction during surgery and after surgery [23]. Presently, it is recommended tricuspid valve excision for right-sided IE in IDUs [23].

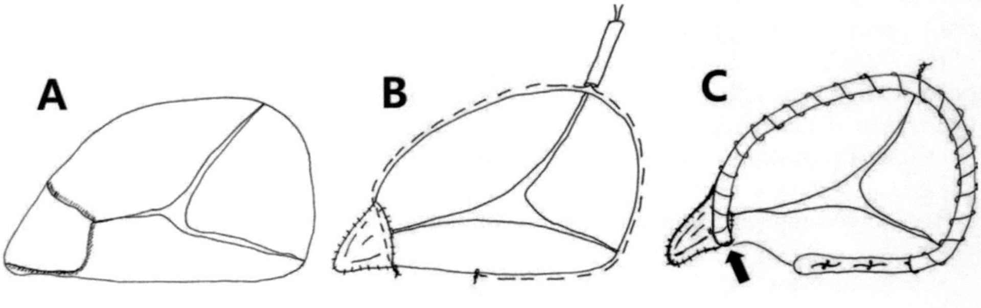

Figure 3.
Operative procedures. (A) After the prolapsed leaflet segments and chordae were excised, the anterior commissural defect was made. (B) The defect was closed with an elliptical pericardial patch of 2.0 × 1.0 cm size. An adjustable DeVega-type annuloplasty using two continuous 5–0 Polypropylene sutures was performed to select an appropriate-size ring for complete leaflet coaptation. (C) A 26-mm Edward MC3 ring was placed using two interrupted, pledgeted 2–0 Dacron sutures and two continuous 3–0 polypropylene sutures. The anterior horn of the rigid ring (black arrow) was sutured to the medial end of the patch. NOTE: every figure specifies this sentence beginning: From Kim et al. [83]. It is an open access article distributed under the terms of the Creative Commons Attribution License (http://creativecommons.org/licenses/by/2.0), which permits unrestricted use, distribution, and reproduction in any medium, provided the original work is properly credited.

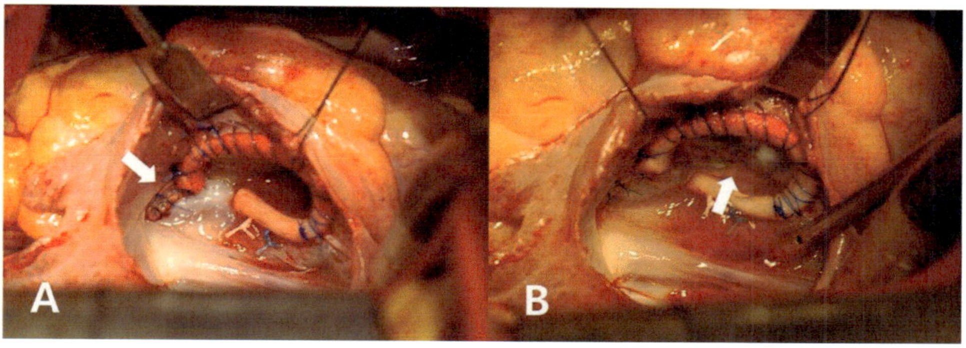

Figure 4.
Operative findings. (A) The anterior commissure defect was closed with a patch (white arrow) and a rigid ring was placed along the functional valve opening. (B) The valve leaflets showed complete coaptation (white arrow) on saline test. NOTE: every figure specifies this sentence beginning: From Kim et al. [83]. It is an open access article distributed under the terms of the Creative Commons Attribution License (http://creativecommons.org/licenses/by/2.0), which permits unrestricted use, distribution, and reproduction in any medium, provided the original work is properly credited.

Valve replacement in IDUs is correlated with greater risk for recurrent infection and redo surgery (re-operation) [81]. It seems that mechanical prostheses and xenografts have similar outcomes [16]. However, recurrence of IE is mainly unchanged for mechanical and bioprosthetic valves [84]. Placement of a bioprosthetic valve may be challenging in case of IDUs with endocarditis considering the low compliance of IDUs for any treatment, risk of recurrent infections, risk of redo surgery, or valve generation. HIV is not a contraindication for surgery having good prognosis after it [85].

An important concern of tricuspid valve surgery is the damage of conduction system, which is higher in TV replacement [81, 86]. For instance, in case of 910 surgeries for tricuspid valve IE, there was higher risk of heart block in TV replacement (16%) versus TV repair (3%, $p < 0.0001$) [86].

Despite of published data supporting the greater risk of morbidity and mortality for multiple valve endocarditis [87], Weymann et al. outlined that single-valve endocarditis or multiple valve involvement have no different operative or postoperative risks [88]. In any type of prosthesis, survival on long-term is similar in any tricuspid valve replacement with prosthesis [89, 90]. Homograft tissue valve may be used after valvectomy mainly with cryopreserved mitral homograft [23].

IDUs have a greater mortality rate in comparison with the general population [91, 92]. However, right-sided IE treated surgically has good outcomes in the early, mid-term, and long-term [86]. Significant risk factors for poor prognosis in IDUs treated surgically are interrelated with the *Staphylococcus aureus* and fungi or polymicrobial IE, late presentation in critical condition, with the vegetation size, and with left-sided IE [93].

Taking into account the current guidelines of The Society of Thoracic Surgeons Workforce on Evidence Based Surgery, European Society of Cardiology, and The European Association for Cardio-Thoracic Surgery, the **first line recommendation** (Class Ia) in IE for IDUs is the excision of infected tissue (vegetation) with valve repair. Furthermore, the second line recommendation (Class IIa) is tricuspid valve replacement. ***Bioprosthesis*** is the principal choice in TV replacement in IDUs, because mechanical valve needs long life anticoagulation [16, 23, 39, 81, 94, 95].

A conservative approach is recommended by ***European Society of Cardiology*** in case of IDUs which present greater risk of recurrent infection. When valve replacement is necessary, bioprosthesis decreases the thromboembolism risk with no anticoagulant therapy on long term. On the other side, younger IDUs are disposed

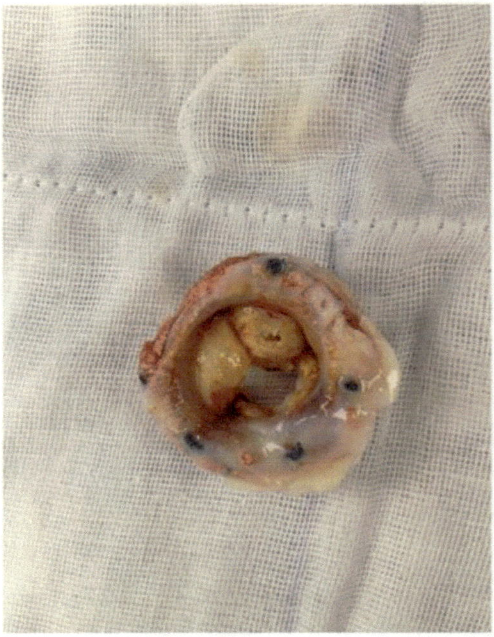

Figure 5.
The damaged bioprosthetic tricuspid valve with vegetations. NOTE: every figure specifies this sentence beginning: From Chen et al. [96]. It is an open access article distributed under the terms of the Creative Commons Attribution License (http://creativecommons.org/licenses/by/4.0/), which permits unrestricted use, distribution, and reproduction in any medium, provided you give appropriate credit to the original author(s) and the source, provide a link to the Creative Commons license, and indicate if changes were made.

to redo surgery or re-operation either because of recurrent infection or valve degeneration (**Figure 5**) [16, 96]. Moreover, valvectomy is the last choice to valve repair or valve replacement in IDUs with greater risk of recurrent infection. The valvectomy technique eludes the use of prosthetic material but is limited by residual severe tricuspid regurgitation with right heart failure. Published data supports this technique because of its long-term survival after complete valvectomy. For instance, one study of Gaca et al. reports tricuspid valvectomy as first choice only in 66 cases from 910 patients (7.3%) [86].

Recurrence of IE is characteristically for IDUs [23, 97]. However, the best indication and timing of surgery are debatable [98]. Prognosis of IE in IDUs has good outcomes with mortality <5% [23]. Right-sided IE has a good prognosis with lower in-hospital mortality. As well, right-sided IE has a lower morbidity and mortality with better prognosis than left-sided IE but with greater early mortality rate [11, 21, 99]. Higher mortality in IDUs with right-sided IE is associated with vegetations >20 mm, fungal endocarditis, bacteremia, and older age [4, 13, 21, 59]. To sum up, the early and complete surgical debridement of infected tissue together with microbial therapy assures a good prognosis on long term [88].

6. Conclusions

Right-sided IE is the primarily disease that affects IDUs and patients with congenital heart diseases [16]. Diagnostic findings comprise fever and respiratory symptoms [16]. In the main part of cases, *S. aureus* is responsible pathogen [16]. For IDUs with IE, optimal treatment strategies lack a general consensus. Majority of strategies are applied based on the team experience and the patient. Furthermore, this absence of evidence-based guidelines highlights that any IE should be managed by an "Endocarditis Team" [86]. Surgery is a choice only for difficult evolution, failure of medical therapy, or recurrent septic emboli to the lungs or paradoxical emboli [16].

Conflict of interest

There are no disclosures.

Author details

Moldovan Horatiu[1,2,3]*, Adrian Molnar[4,5], Victor Costache[6] and Ecaterina Bontas[7]

1 Faculty of Medicine, University Titu Maiorescu, Bucharest, Romania

2 Faculty of Science and Engineering in Biomaterials, University POLITEHNICA of Bucharest, Bucharest, Romania

3 Department of Cardiovascular Surgery, Sanador Clinical Hospital, Bucharest, Romania

4 Department of Cardiovascular Surgery, University of Medicine and Pharmacy, Cluj-Napoca, Romania

5 Department of Cardiovascular Surgery, Heart Institute "Niculae Stancioiu", Cluj-Napoca, Romania

6 Department of Cardiovascular and Thoracic Surgery, POLISANO Hospital, Sibiu, Romania

7 Department of Cardiology, Emergency Institute for Cardiovascular Diseases, Bucharest, Romania

*Address all correspondence to: horatiu.moldovan@sanador.ro

References

[1] Baddour LM, Wilson WR, Bayer AS, Fowler VG Jr, Tleyjeh IM, Rybak MJ, et al. Infective Endocarditis in Adults: Diagnosis, Antimicrobial Therapy, and Management of Complications: A Scientific Statement for Healthcare Professionals From the American Heart Association. Circulation. 2015;**132**(15):1435-1486. DOI: 10.1161/CIR.0000000000000296

[2] Gordon RJ, Lowy FD. Bacterial infections in drug users. The New England Journal of Medicine. 2005;**353**:1945-1954

[3] Miró JM, del Río A, Mestres CA. Infective endocarditis in intravenous drug abusers and HIV-1 infected patients. Infectious Disease Clinics of North America. 2002;**16**:273-295

[4] Miro JM, del Rio A, Mestres CA. Infective endocarditis and cardiac surgery in intravenous drug abusers and HIV-1 infected patients. Cardiology Clinics. 2003;**9**:167-184. DOI: 10.1016/S0733-8651(03)00025-0

[5] Shrestha NK, Jue J, Hussain ST, Jerry JM, et al. Injection drug use and outcomes after surgical intervention for infective endocarditis. The Annals of Thoracic Surgery. 2015;**100**:875-882. DOI: 10.1016/j.athoracsur.2015.03.019

[6] Frontera JA, Gradon JD. Right-side endocarditis in injection drug users: Review of proposed mechanisms of pathogenesis. Clinical Infectious Diseases. 2000;**30**(2):374-379

[7] Starakis I, Mazokopakis EE. Injecting illicit substances epidemic and infective endocarditis. Infectious Disorders Drug Targets. 2010;**10**(1):22-26

[8] Ronan MV, Herzig SJ. Hospitalizations related to opioid abuse/dependence and associated serious infections increased sharply, 2002-2012. Health Affairs (Millwood). 1 May 2016;**35**(5):832-837. DOI: 10.1377/hlthaff.2015.1424

[9] Wurcel AG, Anderson JE, Chui KK, et al. Increasing infectious endocarditis admissions among young people who inject drugs. Open Forum Infectious Diseases. 2016;**3**:ofw157. DOI: 10.1093/ofid/ofw157 9

[10] Hartman L, Barnes E, Bachmann L, Schafer K, Lovato J, Files DC. Opiate injection-associated infective endocarditis in the southeastern United States. The American Journal of the Medical Sciences. 2016;**352**:603-608. DOI: 10.1016/j.amjms.2016.08.010

[11] Ortiz-Bautista C, Lopez J, Garcia-Granja PE, Sevilla T, Vilacosta I, Sarria C, et al. Current profile of infective endocarditis in intravenous drug users: The prognostic relevance of the valves involved. International Journal of Cardiology. 2015;**187**:472-474

[12] Substance Abuse and Mental Health Services Administration. Results from the 2013 National Survey on Drug Use and Health: Summary of National Findings. Rockville: (NSDUH Series H-48, HHS Publication No. SMA 14-4863) Substance Abuse and Mental Health Services Administration; 2014

[13] Otome O, Guy S, Tramontana A, Lane G, Karunajeewa H. A retrospective review: Significance of vegetation size in injection drug users with right-sided infective endocarditis. Heart, Lung & Circulation. 2016;**25**(5):466-470

[14] Yamashita S, Noma K, Kuwata G, Miyoshi K, Honaga K. Infective endocarditis at the tricuspid valve following central venous catheterization. Journal of Anesthesia. 2005;**19**(1):84-87

[15] Armstrong ML, DeBoer S, Cetta F. Infective endocarditis after body art: A

review of the literature and concerns. The Journal of Adolescent Health. 2008;**43**(3):217-225

[16] Habib G, Lancellotti P, Antunes MJ, Bongiorni MG, Casalta JP, Del Zotti F, et al. ESC guidelines for the management of infective endocarditis: The task force for the management of infective endocarditis of the European Society of Cardiology (ESC). Endorsed by: European Association for Cardio-Thoracic Surgery (EACTS), the European Association of Nuclear Medicine (EANM). European Heart Journal. 2015;**36**(44):3075-3128

[17] Chan P, Ogilby J, Segal B. Tricuspid valve endocarditis. American Heart Journal. 1989;**117**(5):1140-1146

[18] Murdoch DR, Corey GR, Hoen B, Miró JM, Fowler VG Jr, Bayer AS, et al. International collaboration on endocarditis-prospective cohort study (ICE-PCS) investigators. Clinical presentation, etiology, and outcome of infective endocarditis in the 21st century: the international collaboration on endocarditis-prospective cohort study. Archives of Internal Medicine. 2009;**169**(5):463-473

[19] Crane LR, Levine DP, Zervos MJ, et al. Bacteremia in narcotic addicts at the Detroit Medical Centre. Microbiology, epidemiology, risk factors and empiric therapy. Reviews of Infectious Diseases. 1986;**8**:364-373

[20] Oylumlu M et al. Both-sided native valve endocarditis in an intravenous drug misuser. BML Case Reports. 2013;**2013**:bcr2013201980. DOI: 10.1136/bcr-2013-201980

[21] Moss R, Munt B. Injection drug use and right sided endocarditis. Heart. 2003;**89**:577-581

[22] Mathew J, Addai T, Anand A, Morrobel A, Maheshwari P, Freels S. Clinical features, site of involvement, bacteriologic findings, and outcome of infective endocarditis in intravenous drug users. Archives of Internal Medicine. 1995;**155**(15):1641-1648

[23] Akinosoglou K, Apostolakis E, Koutsogiannis N, Leivaditis V, Gogos CA. Right-sided infective endocarditis: Surgical management. European Journal of Cardio-Thoracic Surgery. 2012 Sep;**42**(3):470-479. DOI: 10.1093/ejcts/ezs084

[24] Faber M, Frimodt-Møller N, Espersen F, Skinhøj P, Rosdahl V. *Staphylococcus aureus* endocarditis in Danish intravenous drug users: High proportion of left sided endocarditis. Scandinavian Journal of Infectious Diseases. 1995;**27**:483-487

[25] Hecht SR, Berger M. Right-sided endocarditis in intravenous drug users: Prognostic features in 102 episodes. Annals of Internal Medicine. 1992;**117**:560-566

[26] Chu VH, Park LP, Athan E, Delahaye F, Freiberger T, Lamas C, et al. Association between surgical indications, operative risk, and clinical outcome in infective endocarditis: A prospective study from the international collaboration on endocarditis. Circulation. 2015;**131**:131-140

[27] Ternhag A, Cederstrom A, Torner A, Westling K. A nationwide cohort study of mortality risk and long-term prognosis in infective endocarditis in Sweden. PLoS One. 2013;**8**:e67519

[28] Nishimura RA, Otto CM, Bonow RO, et al. 2014 AHA/ACC guideline for the management of patients with valvular heart disease: Executive summary: A report of the American college of cardiology/ American heart association task force on practice guidelines. Circulation. 2014;**129**:2440-2492. DOI: 10.1161/ CIR.0000000000000029

[29] Shih CJ, Chu H, Chao PW, Lee YJ, Kuo SC, Li SY, et al. Long-term clinical

outcome of major adverse cardiac events in survivors of infective endocarditis: A nationwide population-based study. Circulation. 2014;**130**:1684-1691

[30] Kaushik KS, Kapila K, Praharaj AK. Shooting up: The interface of microbial infections and drug abuse. Journal of Medical Microbiology. 2011;**60**(Pt 4):408-422. DOI: 10.1099/jmm.0.027540-0

[31] Yong MS, Coffey S, Prendergast BD, Marasco SF, Zimmet AD, McGiffin DC, et al. Surgical management of tricuspid valve endocarditis in the current era: A review. International Journal of Cardiology. 2016;**202**:44-48. DOI: 10.1016/j.ijcard.2015.08.211

[32] Mah MW, Shafran SD. Polymicrobial endocarditis with eight pathogens in an intravenous drug abuser. Scandinavian Journal of Infectious Diseases. 1990;**22**(6):735-737

[33] Oh S, Havlen PR, Hussain N. A case of polymicrobial endocarditis caused by anaerobic organisms in an injection drug user. Journal of General Internal Medicine. 2005;**20**(10):958

[34] Silpa M, D'Angelo J. *Eikenella corrodens* infections in drug abusers. Annals of Internal Medicine. 1980;**92**(6):871

[35] Raucher B, Dobkin J, Mandel L, Edberg S, Levi M, Miller M. Occult polymicrobial endocarditis with *Haemophilus parainfluenzae* in intravenous drug abusers. The American Journal of Medicine. 1989;**86**(2):169-172

[36] Deutscher M, Perlman DC. Why some injection drug users lick their needles: A preliminary survey. The International Journal on Drug Policy. 2008;**19**(4):342-345

[37] Lee MR, Chang SA, Choi SH, Lee GY, Kim EK, Peck KR, et al. Clinical features of right-sided infective endocarditis occurring in non-drug users. Journal of Korean Medical Science. 2014;**29**(6):776-781

[38] Kaiser SP, Melby SJ, Zierer A, Schuessler RB, Moon MR, Moazami N, et al. Long-term outcomes in valve replacement surgery for infective endocarditis. The Annals of Thoracic Surgery. 2007;**83**:30-35

[39] Rabkin DG, Mokadam NA, Miller DW, Goetz RR, Verrier ED, Aldea GS. Long-term outcome for the surgical treatment of infective endocarditis with a focus on intravenous drug users. The Annals of Thoracic Surgery. 2012;**93**:51-57. DOI: 10.1016/j.athoracsur.2011.08.016

[40] Wilson LE, Thomas DL, Astemborski J, et al. Prospective study of infective endocarditis among injection drug users. The Journal of Infectious Diseases. 2002;**185**:1761-1766

[41] Chu VH, Sexton DJ, Cabell CH, Reller LB, Pappas PA, Singh RK, et al. Repeat infective endocarditis: Differentiating relapse from reinfection. Clinical Infectious Diseases. 2005;**41**:406-409

[42] Sousa C, Botelho C, Rodrigues D, Azeredo J, Oliveira R. Infective endocarditis in intravenous drug abusers: An update. European Journal of Clinical Microbiology & Infectious Diseases. 2012;**31**:2905-2910

[43] Baraki H, Saito S, Al Ahmad A, et al. Surgical treatment for isolated tricuspid valve endocarditis- long-term follow-up at a single institution. Circulation Journal. 2013;**77**:2032-2037. DOI: 10.1253/circj.CJ-12-1364

[44] Lamas CC, Eykyn SJ. Blood culture negative endocarditis: Analysis of 63 cases presenting over 25 years. Heart. 2003;**89**(3):258-262

[45] Lowes JA, Hamer J, Williams G, Houang E, Tabaqchali S, Shaw EJ, et al.

10 years of infective endocarditis at St. Bartholomew's hospital: Analysis of clinical features and treatment in relation to prognosis and mortality. Lancet. 1980;**1**(8160):133-136

[46] Cabell CH, Abrutyn E, Fowler VG Jr, et al. Use of surgery in patients with native valve infective endocarditis: Results from the International Collaboration on Endocarditis Merged Database. American Heart Journal. 2005;**150**:1092-1098. DOI: 10.1016/j.ahj.2005.03.057

[47] Cicalini S, Forcina G, De Rosa FG. Infective endocarditis in patients with human immunodeficiency virus infection. The Journal of Infection. 2001;**42**:267-271

[48] Levine DP, Crane LR, Zervos MJ. Bacteremia in narcotic addicts at the Detroit Medical Center. II. Infectious endocarditis: A prospective comparative study. Reviews of Infectious Diseases. 1986;**8**(3):374-396

[49] Moreillon P, Que YA. Infective endocarditis. Lancet. 2004;**363**:139-149. DOI: 10.1016/S0140-6736(03)15266-X

[50] Wanahita A, Goldsmith EA, Musher DM, Clarridge JE 3rd, Rubio J, Krishnan B, et al. Interaction between human polymorphonuclear leukocytes and *Streptococcus milleri* group bacteria. The Journal of Infectious Diseases. 2002;**185**(1):85-90

[51] Young KA, Allaker RP, Hardie JM, Whiley RA. Interactions between *Eikenella corrodens* and '*Streptococcus milleri*-group' organisms: Possible mechanisms of pathogenicity in mixed infections. Antonie Van Leeuwenhoek. 1996;**69**(4):371-373

[52] Bottone EJ, Kittick J Jr, Schneierson SS. Isolation of bacillus HB-1 from human clinical sources. American Journal of Clinical Pathology. 1973;**59**(4):5606

[53] Cahill TJ, Prendergast BD. Infective endocarditis. Lancet. 2016;**387**(10021):882

[54] Bayer AS, Bolger AF, Taubert KA, Wilson W, Steckelberg J, Karchmer AW, et al. Diagnosis and management of infective endocarditis and its complications. Circulation. 1998;**9**:2936-2948. DOI: 10.1161/01.CIR.98.25.2936

[55] Yuan SM. Right-sided infective endocarditis: Recent epidemiologic changes. International Journal of Clinical and Experimental Medicine. 2014;**7**(1):199-218

[56] Welton DE, Young JB, Gentry WO. Recurrent infective endocarditis. Analysis of predisposing factors and clinical features. The American Journal of Medicine. 1979;**66**(6):932-938

[57] Bai Z, Hou J, Ren W, Guo Y. Diagnosis and surgical treatment for isolated tricuspid Libman-Sacks endocarditis: A rare case report and literatures review. Journal of Cardiothoracic Surgery. 2015;**10**:93. DOI: 10.1186/s13019-015-0302-1

[58] Leitman M, Dreznik Y, Tyomkin V, et al. Vegetation size in patients with infective endocarditis. European Heart Journal Cardiovascular Imaging. 2012;**13**(4):330-338

[59] Martín-Dávila P, Navas E, Fortún J, et al. Analysis of mortality and risk factors associated with native valve endocarditis in drug users: The importance of vegetation size. American Heart Journal. 2005;**150**(5):1099-1106

[60] Cahill TJ, Baddour LM, Habib G, Hoen B, Salaun E, Pettersson GB, et al. Challenges in infective endocarditis. Journal of the American College of Cardiology. 2017;**69**(3):325-344. DOI: 10.1016/j.jacc.2016.10.066

[61] Habib G, Badano L, Tribouilloy C, Vilacosta I, Zamorano JL, Galderisi M, et al. Recommendations for the practice of echocardiography in infective endocarditis. European Journal of Echocardiography. 2010;**11**(2):202-219

[62] Winslow T, Foster E, Adams JR, Schiller NB. Pulmonary valve endocarditis: Improved diagnosis with biplane transesophageal echocardiography. Journal of the American Society of Echocardiography. 1992;**5**:206-210

[63] Durack DT, Lukes AS, Bright DK. New criteria for diagnosis of infective endocarditis: Utilization of specific echocardiographic findings. Duke endocarditis service. The American Journal of Medicine. 1994;**96**(3):200-209

[64] Li JS, Sexton DJ, Mick N, Nettles R, Fowler VGJ, Ryan T, et al. Proposed modifications to the Duke criteria for the diagnosis of infective endocarditis. Clinical Infectious Diseases. 2000;**30**:633-638. DOI: 10.1086/313753

[65] Liu YW, Tsai WC, Lin CC, Hsu CH, Li WT, Lin LJ, et al. Usefulness of real-time three-dimensional echocardiography for diagnosis of infective endocarditis. Scandinavian Cardiovascular Journal. 2009;**43**:318-323

[66] Westling K, Aufwerber E, Ekdahl C, Friman G, Gardlund B, Julander I, et al. Swedish guidelines for diagnosis and treatment of infective endocarditis. Scandinavian Journal of Infectious Diseases. 2007;**39**:929-946

[67] Bisbe J, Miro JM, Latorre X, Moreno A, Mallolas J, Gatell JM, et al. Disseminated candidiasis in addicts who use brown heroin: Report of 83 cases and review. Clinical Infectious Diseases. 1992;**15**:910-923

[68] Ribera E, Gomez-Jimenez J, Cortes E, del Valle O, Planes A, Gonzalez-Alujas T, et al. Effectiveness of cloxacillin with and without gentamicin in short-term therapy for right-sided *Staphylococcus aureus* endocarditis. A randomized, controlled trial. Annals of Internal Medicine. 1996;**125**:969-974

[69] Fowler VG Jr, Boucher HW, Corey GR, Abrutyn E, Karchmer AW, Rupp ME, et al. Daptomycin versus standard therapy for bacteremia and endocarditis caused by *Staphylococcus aureus*. The New England Journal of Medicine. 2006;**355**:653-665. DOI: 10.1056/NEJMoa053783

[70] Haber PS, Demirkol A, Lange K, Murnion B. Management of injecting drug users admitted to hospital. Lancet. 2009;**374**:1284-1293

[71] Arbulu A, Holmes RJ, Asfaw I. Surgical treatment of intractable right-sided infective endocarditis in drug addicts: 25 years experience. The Journal of Heart Valve Disease. 1993;**2**:129-137; discussion 138-9

[72] Carozza A, De Santo LS, Romano G, Della Corte A, Ursomando F, Scardone M, et al. Infective endocarditis in intravenous drug abusers: Patterns of presentation and longterm outcomes of surgical treatment. The Journal of Heart Valve Disease. 2006;**15**(1):125-131

[73] Levison ME, Kaye D, Mandell GL, Hook EW. Characteristics of patients with multiple episodes of bacterial endocarditis. Journal of the American Medical Association. 1970;**211**(8):1355-1357

[74] Miljeteig I, Skrede S, Langorgen J, Haaverstad R, Josendal O, Sjursen H, et al. Should patients who use illicit drugs be offered a second heart-valve replacement? Tidsskrift for den Norske laegeforening: tidsskrift for praktisk medicinny raekke. 2013;**133**:977-980

[75] Bonow RO, Carabello BA, Kanu C, et al. ACC/AHA 2006 Guidelines for

the management of patients with valvular heart disease. A report of the American college of cardiology/American heart association task force on practice guidelines. Circulation. 2006;**114**(5):e84-e231

[76] Musci M, Siniawski H, Pasic M, Grauhan O, Weng Y, Meyer R, et al. Surgical treatment of right-sided active infective endocarditis with or without involvement of the left heart: 20-year single center experience. European Journal of Cardio-Thoracic Surgery. 2007;**32**:118-125. DOI: 10.1016/j.ejcts.2007.02.034

[77] Sohail MR, Uslan DZ, Khan AH, Friedman PA, Hayes DL, Wilson WR, et al. Infective endocarditis complicating permanent pacemaker and implantable cardioverter-defibrillator infection. Mayo Clinic Proceedings. 2008;**83**:46-53

[78] Chrissoheris MP, Libertin C, Ali RG, Ghantous A, Bekui A, Donohue T. Endocarditis complicating central venous catheter bloodstream infections: A unique form of health care associated endocarditis. Clinical Cardiology. 2009;**32**:E48-E54

[79] Denk K, Vahl CF. Infective endocarditis: Considerations regarding optimal timing for surgical treatment. Herz. 2009;**34**(3):198-205. DOI: 10.1007/s00059-009-3232-7

[80] Gutierrez-Martin MA, Galvez-Aceval J, Araji OA. Indications for surgery and operative techniques in infective endocarditis in the present day. Infectious Disorders Drug Targets. 2010;**10**(1):32-46

[81] Dawood MY, Cheema FH, Ghoreishi M, et al. Contemporary outcomes of operations for tricuspid valve infective endocarditis. The Annals of Thoracic Surgery. 2015;**99**:539-546. DOI: 10.1016/j.athoracsur.2014.08.069

[82] Yanagawa B, Elbatarny M, Verma S, Hill S, Mazine A, Puskas JD, et al. Surgical management of tricuspid valve infective endocarditis: A systematic review and meta-analysis. The Annals of Thoracic Surgery. 2018;**106**(3):708-714. DOI: 10.1016/j.athoracsur.2018.04.012

[83] Kim JH, Kim KH, JB1 C, Kuh JH. Commissuroplasty for the anterior commissure defect caused by tricuspid valve endocarditis using patch closure and modified placement of a rigid ring. Journal of Cardiothoracic Surgery. 2014;**9**:36. DOI: 10.1186/1749-8090-9-36

[84] Grover FL, Cohen DJ, Oprian C, Henderson WG, Sethi G, Hammermeister KE. Determinants of the occurrence of and survival from prosthetic valve endocarditis. Experience of the Veterans affairs cooperative study on valvular heart disease. The Journal of Thoracic and Cardiovascular Surgery. 1994;**108**:207-214

[85] Mestres CA, Chuquiure JE, Claramonte X, Muñoz J, Benito N, Castro MA, et al. Long-term results after cardiac surgery in patients infected with the human immunodeficiency virus type-1. European Journal of Cardio-Thoracic Surgery. 2003;**23**:1007-1016

[86] Gaca JG, Sheng S, Daneshmand M, et al. Current outcomes for tricuspid valve infective endocarditis surgery in North America. The Annals of Thoracic Surgery. 2013;**96**:1374-1381. DOI: 10.1016/j.athoracsur.2013.05.046

[87] Kim N, Lazar JM, Cunha BA, Liao W, Minnaganti V. Multi-valvular endocarditis. Clinical Microbiology and Infection. 2000;**6**:207-212

[88] Weymann A, Borst T, Popov AF, Sabashnikov A, Bowles C, Schmack B, et al. Surgical treatment of infective endocarditis in active intravenous drug users: A justified procedure? Journal of Cardiothoracic Surgery. 2014;**9**:58. DOI: 10.1186/1749-8090-9-58

[89] Filsoufi F, Anyanwu AC, Salzberg SP, et al. Long-term outcomes of tricuspid valve replacement in the current era. The Annals of Thoracic Surgery. 2005;**80**:845-850. DOI: 10.1016/j.athoracsur.2004.12.019

[90] Chang BC, Lim SH, Yi G, et al. Long-term clinical results of tricuspid valve replacement. The Annals of Thoracic Surgery. 2006;**81**:1317-1323, discussion 1323-4. DOI: 10.1016/j.athoracsur.2005.11.005

[91] Joe GW, Simpson DD. Mortality rates among opioid addicts in a longitudinal study. American Journal of Public Health. 1987;**77**:347-348

[92] Frischer M, Goldberg D, Rahman M, Berney L. Mortality and survival among a cohort of drug injectors in Glasgow, 1982-1994. Addiction. 1997;**92**:419-427

[93] Zhang L, Gao CQ, Jiang SL, Ren CL. Surgical treatment of isolated right-sided infective endocarditis. Zhonghua Wai Ke Za Zhi. 2010;**48**(5):342-344

[94] Gottardi R, Bialy J, Devyatko E, et al. Midterm follow-up of tricuspid valve reconstruction due to active infective endocarditis. The Annals of Thoracic Surgery. 2007;**84**:1943-1948. DOI: 10.1016/j.athoracsur.2007.04.116

[95] Tarola CL, Losenno KL, Chu MW. Complex tricuspid valve repair for infective endocarditis: Leaflet augmentation, chordae and annular reconstruction. Multimedia Manual of Cardiothoracic Surgery. 2015;**2015**

[96] Chen Q, Cao H, Lu H, Qiu ZH, He JJ. Bioprosthetic tricuspid valve endocarditis caused by *Acinetobacter baumannii* complex, a case report and brief review of the literature. Journal of Cardiothoracic Surgery. 2015;**10**:149. DOI: 10.1186/s13019-015-0377-8

[97] Fayad G, Modine T, Lions C, Polge AS, Azzaoui R, Larrue B, et al. Conservative surgical treatment for active infective tricuspid valve endocarditis according to the "clover technique". The Heart Surgery Forum. 2008;**11**(2):E120-E126. DOI: 10.1532/HSF98.20071188

[98] Pang PY, Sin YK, Lim CH, Tan TE, Lim SL, Chao VT, et al. Surgical management of infective endocarditis: An analysis of early and late outcomes. European Journal of Cardio-Thoracic Surgery. 2015;**47**(5):826-832. DOI: 10.1093/ejcts/ezu281

[99] Ortiz C, López J, García H, Sevilla T, Revilla A, Vilacosta I, et al. Clinical classification and prognosis of isolated right-sided infective endocarditis. Medicine (Baltimore). 2014;**93**(27):e137

Chapter 5

Infective Endocarditis: Inflammatory Response, Genetic Susceptibility, Oxidative Stress, and Multiple Organ Failure

Pedro Eduardo Alvarado Rubio MD,
Roberto Brugada Molina MD,
Pedro Eduardo Alvarado Ávila MD,
Alejandro González Mora MD and
Cesar Augusto González López MD

Abstract

Infective endocarditis is defined by a focus of infection within the heart. Despite the optimal care, the mortality approaches 30% at 1 year, so the care for this type of patients represents a challenge to improve the result in your care. The challenges in this clinical entity have several aspects such as the diversity of germs that cause endocarditis, and the most important epidemiologically has generated resistance to antimicrobial treatment along with the possibility of apoptosis in their host-germ interaction. The immunogenetic susceptibility to host infection is discussed, which represents a deep area of research. Inflammation, local and systemic, is complex, with the genesis of reactive oxygen species, which are harmful when the antioxidant defenses are exceeded, causing the break in the mitochondrial electron transport chain with the fall in energy genesis, multiple organ failure, and death. Both at the cellular level and in the mitochondria, possible therapeutic targets are also commented.

Keywords: infective endocarditis, *Staphylococcus aureus*, single nucleotide polymorphism (SNP), inflammatory response, reactive oxygen species (ROS), oxidative stress, multiple organ failure (MOF)

1. Introduction

In this chapter we will analyze the physiopathological changes involved in the inflammatory response of the septic process in infective endocarditis [IE] that culminate with cellular damage and the generation of organic failures; morphological changes, cellular biology, biochemistry, immunology, and genetic vulnerability, which together are called "pathobiology," are the substrate of clinical manifestations of this serious disease, which requires a multidisciplinary group of experts (cardiologists, infectologists, surgeons, intensivists) to optimize therapeutic approach. IE is defined as a severe multisystem disease, which results from an infection, often bacterial, that initially affects the endocardial surface of the heart [1]. The epidemiological pattern has changed over time [2–4]. The incidence has increased in recent years to 5–10 cases per 100,000 inhabitants [2], due to the fact of a greater number of predisposing factors such as the use of permanent cardiovascular devices, invasion with intravenous catheters in critical care units, and hemodialysis treatments, in addition to having greater accessibility to diagnostic tools. From the etiological point of view, *Staphylococcus aureus* (*S. aureus*) is predominant as a causal germ [5, 6]. The clinical course of a patient with IE depends on the inflammatory response, since it is variable; it also depends on the germ and the response of the patient to infection with varying degrees of hemodynamic and metabolic compromise [7–9]. We emphasize the current trend of the search for organic failures associated to the septic processes for their identification and stratification and therapeutic approach [10]. Given the characteristics of the disease, IE has a high mortality that goes from 20 to 30% in the reported series [2, 11]; it is noteworthy that the evolution toward septic shock has been documented in 30% [12], considering this complication as an independent variable of poor prognosis [13].

2. Epidemiology of infective endocarditis

The pathogenesis and the prognosis of IE can be simply described in a general way as the interaction between the host and the germ; however, these factors are not independent and are very importantly linked both in the susceptibility characteristics of the host (advanced age, higher prevalence of comorbid conditions, and exposure to health care) to survive or not to an infectious state, as of the characteristics of the germ involved. To reduce the incidence of IE and improve its outcome, epidemiological studies can provide valuable information on contemporary and modifiable risks to modify their morbidity and mortality [14].

The incidence of hospital discharge diagnoses for drug dependence combined with IE increased more than twelvefold from 0.2 to 2.7 per 100,000 persons per year over this 6-year period. Correspondingly, hospital costs for these patients increased eighteenfold, from $1.1 million in 2010 to $22.2 million in 2015 [15].

In another study also conducted in the USA, using a national sample of hospitalized patients from 1998 to 2009 with focus on IE showed an increase in the use of intracardiac devices from 13.3 to 18.9%. In cases with pathogens identified, *S. aureus* was the most common, increasing from 37.6% in 1998 to 49.3% in 2009, 53.3% of which were methicillin-resistant *Staphylococcus aureus* (MRSA) [16]. The above can give us an idea of the economic and assistance impact of treating patients with severe sepsis such as IE. It is an infection inside the organ that is responsible for distributing blood to practically the whole organism.

The evolution of an inflammatory process plus infection frequently occurs with clinical manifestations unspecified such as fever or hypothermia, tachycardia, tachypnea, or abnormal white blood cell count, progressing to septic shock and acute organ failure [17].

Epidemiological data of more than five decades tell us that *S. aureus* is the most important causal agent of IE [4]; so in the development of systemic inflammation that is generated by the host-germ interaction, we will consider the *S. aureus* as the best example of IE due to its virulence and an emergent property that we know as resistance to antibiotics, sophisticated defense mechanisms, and the ability to cause apoptosis in cells when it is alive inside the cell. The interaction of *S. aureus*-host allows us to develop in a substantive way, on one hand, the importance of the virulence of the germ and, on the other, the defense mechanisms of the host, showing how the inflammation is generated and amplified to offer a step to oxidative stress. It is important to mention that other agents can cause IE such as streptococci and fungi.

3. *Staphylococcus aureus*

S. aureus is a Gram-positive coccus with a diameter of 0.5–1.5 μm, grouped as single cells, in pairs, tetrads, short chains, or forming a conglomerate in a cluster of grapes. This microorganism was first described in the year 1880, in Aberdeen, Scotland, by the surgeon Alexander Ágoston. The name comes from the Greek σταφυλόκοκκος, which is composed of the terms "staphylé," meaning cluster, and coccus, meaning grain or grape, and from the Latin "aureus" which means golden, that is to say "cluster of golden grapes."

They are non-motile bacteria, not sporulated, with no capsule (although there are some strains that develop a slime capsule); they are facultative anaerobes. Most staphylococci produce catalase (enzyme capable of dismutating hydrogen peroxide in $H_2O + O_2$), characteristic that is used to differentiate its sort from others like *Streptococcus* and *Enterococcus*. In 1961, the first report was made on the existence of a methicillin-resistant *Staphylococcus aureus* [18].

3.1 *Staphylococcus aureus* and endothelial cell

S. aureus is a pathogen that causes significant morbidity and mortality worldwide [2]. It is the leading pathogen associated with life-threatening bloodstream infections [19].

Although *S. aureus* is mainly known as an extracellular pathogen, it has been shown to invade and survive within endothelial cells, both within vacuoles and free in the cytoplasm, which implies that the bacteria can escape from the phagolysosome. *S. aureus* tends to infect endovascular tissue. It is believed that this ability contributes to causing a persistent endovascular infection with endothelial destruction.

3.2 Endothelial cell and *Staphylococcus aureus* ingestion

On the other hand, the death of endothelial cells after the invasion of *S. aureus* occurs at least in part by apoptosis, as demonstrated by DNA fragmentation and changes in nuclear morphology. Apoptotic changes are observed as early as 1 h after infection of endothelial cells [18]; they are considered to function as nonprofessional phagocytes, being able to ingest *S. aureus* [20, 21] following the adhesion of this to endothelial cell monolayers; invasion can occur through ingestion by endothelial cells.

For the internalization of *S. aureus*, adherence seems to be necessary, since the use of the phagocytosis inhibitor cytochalasin D prevented apoptosis. Studies show that living intracellular *S. aureus* induces apoptosis of endothelial cells and that this depends on a factor associated with viable organisms, since dead *S. aureus* (by ultraviolet light) also internalized does not induce it [18]. The process has been observed through electron transmission micrographs of bovine aortic endothelial cell monolayers infected with *S. aureus*, showing phagocytosis following a sequence of events: (I) adhesion of *S. aureus* to the endothelial cell, (II) formation of cup-shaped processes on the surface of the endothelial cell underlying the adherent bacteria, and (III) elongation of the cup and engulfment of bacteria within a phagosome [19].

3.3 Heme prosthetic group and *Staphylococcus aureus*

To colonize a vertebrate host, *S. aureus* requires numerous nutrients, such as the prosthetic group heme. The requirement can be met through two distinct mechanisms: importing exogenous heme through dedicated machinery or synthesizing endogenous heme from own metabolic precursors. These two mechanisms are necessary for a complete virulence of *S. aureus* [22, 23]. Once acquired, heme is used for several cell processes. The intact heme is used as a cofactor for enzymes [24], including cytochromes in the electron transport chain, catalase for the detoxification of reactive oxygen species, and bacterial nitric oxide synthase (bNOS).

Although the *S. aureus* requires heme, its excess is toxic to the germ, so it has a mechanism for hem detoxification through a hem sensor system (HssRS) that induces the expression of a hem regulator transporter (hrtAB) [25]. The suppression of the components of this route affects the virulence of *S. aureus*. This ability to detoxify heme is critical to survive in the host. Also, the synthesis of nitric oxide is important for the bacteria to survive. Bacteria encode genes similar to nitric oxide synthetase in mammals, which leads to the characterization of the nitric oxide synthase hemoprotein (bNOS) [26].

3.4 *Staphylococcus aureus* as a pro-inflammatory agent

The *S. aureus* contains molecules such as peptidoglycan and lipoteichoic acid, potent stimulants for the production of cytosines such as TNF-α, IL-4, IL-6, IL-8, IL-12, IL-1be, growth-regulated oncogene (GRO) alpha, and regulated upon activation, normal T-cell expressed, and secreted (RANTES). RANTES has a chemotactic function to perform leukocyte recruitment to areas of infection in addition to inducing tumor necrosis factor alpha and interleukin 1. Elevated levels can persist for 7–14 days [27]. As we can observe, *S. aureus* activates in a very important way the process of inflammation.

3.5 *Staphylococcus aureus* and blood stream infections in infective endocarditis

Circulatory blood stream infections (positive blood cultures) occur in patients with intravascular prosthetic devices as the most common source of infections related to health care [28]. MRSA was the most frequent pathogen in these types of infections with a consistent increase in the isolates of MRSA [29–31]. In the EU, epidemiological surveillance data on bloodstream infections show a marked variability among the member countries that make up a proportion of *S. aureus* that is resistant to methicillin, ranging from less than 1% to more than 50%. In addition to infections associated with health care, new MRSA strains have emerged in their communities as human pathogens associated with livestock [32].

3.6 Endocardial endothelium and myocardial capillary endothelium

The anatomical and physiological barriers of cardiac protection such as the endothelium can be compromised in its structure when areas of turbulence and injury are generated, producing an area exposed to infection. The intracardiac cavities have a cell layer called endocardial endothelium (EE) that covers the endocardium of the atria, ventricles, and all their anatomical components (papillary muscles, chordae tendineae, and heart valves). The EE acts as an active mechanism of biological heart-blood barrier, since it interacts dynamically with cardiomyocytes allowing direct communication and signaling between both types of cells. This electrochemical communication between the cells of the EE and the cardiomyocytes allows a rapid intracellular electrochemical propagation and amplification of the functional properties of the EE.

Signaling between cardiac endothelial cells (EE and myocardial capillary endothelium) and cardiomyocytes influences cardiac growth, contractile performance, and rhythmicity. The network of Purkinje fibers and the subendocardial neural plexus (parasympathetic nervous system) is immediately below the endocardial endothelium (EE) and participates in the endothelial control of cardiac rhythm. Endothelin-1 (Et-1), nitric oxide (ON), prostaglandins (PGI2), prostacyclin (AI and AII), angiotensin I and II, and vascular endothelial growth factor (VEGF) are involved in these processes.

The endothelium that covers cardiac structures is at the vascular level, the myocardial capillary, and the endocardium; its activation includes changes in the endothelial phenotype as part of the physiological adaptive response to several possible injuries and stressors. The dysfunction of the endothelium implies a deregulated response that is not useful and that can be permanent.

One of the clinical disorders that selectively damage the endocardium and subendocardial interstitial tissue is endocarditis. This entity causes activation of the vascular and endocardial endothelial system, as well as poor adaptation or failure characterized by hemodynamic abnormalities, neurohormonal imbalance, cytokine expression, and endothelial dysfunction [33].

Infective endocarditis is an anatomoclinical entity characterized by microbial infection of the valvular or parietal endothelium or both; it is located predominantly on the left side of the heart, although it can also occur in the right (e.g., endovenous drug), which produces inflammation, exudation, and proliferation of the endocardium. The most characteristic lesion is the vegetation, constituted by an amorphous mass of platelets and fibrin, of variable size, which contains multiple microorganisms and scarce inflammatory cells (fibrinoplaquetary thrombus) [34]. This type of lesions generates metastatic infection in other anatomical territories, for example, the central nervous system, apostematous meningitis, myocarditis, pyelonephritis, and splenic abscesses which are at risk of rupture [35, 36].

4. Clinical manifestations

The clinical manifestations of infective endocarditis are acute rapidly progressive or subacute; the pathophysiological processes of both are explained by immunological and vascular phenomena, such as inflammatory response, mediators of inflammation triggered by a maladaptive response to an infectious process, aggregation of immune complexes, infectious vasculitis, and peripheral microembolism [34, 37]. Depending on the affected cardiac cavity (right/left) or valvular system, the clinical manifestations will be due to the aforementioned processes [38] (**Table 1**).

4.1 Anatomopathological changes

The anatomopathological changes due to the formation of vegetations in the valvular ring and/or in the leaflets cause an anatomical alteration. If this anatomical alteration generated by a vegetation prevents valvular closure, it will be expressed as a murmur of valvular insufficiency and in severe cases such as microembolisms septic and non-septic and cardiac failure [34, 37].

	Patients, %
Sign	
Fever	86–96
New murmur	48
Worsening of old murmur	20
Hematuria	26
Vascular embolic event	17
Splenomegaly	11
Splinter hemorrhages	8
Osler nodes	3
Janeway lesions	5
Roth spots	2
Complication	
Stroke	17–20
Non-stroke embolization	23–33
Heart failure	14–33
Intracardiac abscess	14–20
New conduction abnormality	8
Murdoch et al. [38].	

Table 1.
Clinical signs and complications of infective endocarditis.

4.2 Considerations on the cardiac cavity affected by infective endocarditis

The standard reference to corroborate the clinical diagnosis of IE is transesophageal echocardiography since the transthoracic echocardiogram, even when limited to native valves, decreases the diagnostic probability of IE [39].

Right and left endocarditis are two distinct entities that require different clinical and surgical approaches. The diagnosis of endocarditis on the right side requires a high index of clinical suspicion. It can occur with a history of intravenous drug use, fever, and pulmonary infiltrates, although intravenous drug abuse is also a cause of IE on the left side of the heart [36]. The information provided by echocardiography is of prognostic and therapeutic value.

If the vegetation is <1.0 cm in diameter, it can be expected that antibiotic therapy will resolve the infection; if the size of the vegetation determined by echocardiography is ≥1.0 cm without response to treatment, surgical intervention should be considered [40].

Surgical treatment in IE on the left side of the heart, for example, the mitral valve, is indicated in patients with severe mitral regurgitation, even in the absence of congestive heart failure, with mitral annular abscess, large vegetation >10 mm, uncontrolled sepsis, and multiple embolisms [41]. Mitral valve (MV) replacement has traditionally been considered as the standard treatment for MV endocarditis that does not respond to antibiotic treatment.

However, the pioneering work of Dreyfus et al. surgery for repair of the mitral valve with IE can be performed safely and is often associated with a better outcome compared to mitral valve replacement [42, 43].

5. Role of immunogenetics in the physiopathology of sepsis and infective endocarditis

5.1 Introduction

It has been largely recognized that infective processes have considerably different patient-to-patient behavior in such a way that some patients respond well to the treatment applied and some others end up developing a dysregulated immune response known as sepsis [44], organ failure, and some even die from this process. Infective endocarditis does not escape from this fact. Many variables, such as the virulence of the pathogen and the quality of the treatment applied, among many others, participate in an additive manner to conform the clinical outcomes of infections, and this helps to understand why a patient takes the road of success or failure regarding the control of the septic process. One of the most recent advances in the understanding of the pathophysiology of infective processes, including infective endocarditis, is the demonstration that genetically determined differences in the immune system of individuals are one of these many factors that determine the phenotypic behavior and outcomes. Therefore, the next chapter section is dedicated to explaining the existing evidence of the participation of immunogenetics in the development of infective endocarditis and sepsis.

Recently, the concept of sepsis has been redefined as the result of a better understanding of its pathophysiology, particularly regarding the early activation of pro- and anti-inflammatory immune responses. As the third international consensus definition of sepsis states, sepsis is a life-threatening organ dysfunction caused by a dysregulated host response to an infection [45]. Then, if sepsis is dependent on a dysregulated response, and this response is executed principally by the host immune system, then genetically defined differences between individuals immune system might play a role in the genesis of this syndrome and at least partially explain why some patients take the road of sepsis and some others do not. This hypothesis had long been existed, but it was until 1988 that the theory started gaining scientific evidence of its existence, when Sørensen et al. [46] published what is considered a landmark study with respect to this topic. In this article, the authors studied the genetical influences on the principal causes of nonviolent premature death in the Danish population; to separate them from the environmental influences, they studied a selected group of people that had been adopted early in life. This was extracted from the Danish Adoption Registry and included adoptees that were born between 1924 and 1926. They traced them up and demonstrated that the death of a biologic parent from an infection before the age of 50 resulted in a relative risk of death from infective causes in the adoptees of 4.5. Since this publication, a great number of studies have been conducted in an attempt to define the specific genetic variations that determine these differences in outcome. This task has resulted complex; as both pro- and anti-inflammatory responses contribute to the outcome of septic processes, all genes encoding effector proteins in the biochemical pathways of the inflammatory response to infection are potential candidates to determine the genetical background responsible for the interindividual differences aforementioned [47].

5.1.1 The study of single nucleotide polymorphism associations with sepsis and IE outcomes.

The most studied specific type of genetic anomaly regarding to sepsis susceptibility is the single nucleotide polymorphism (SNP); therefore, the largest body of evidence comes from the study of this type of genetic variations. SNPs are defined as frequent (occurring in >1% of the population) variations in the human DNA sequence [48] and consist in the exchange of a single base pair for another in a specific location in the DNA sequence. They may occur within the exonic (coding) or intronic (noncoding) region of the gene and can have different consequences which include alteration of expression or structure of proteins and enzymes, introduction of an alternative translation initiation codon or stop codon, and destabilization of exonic mRNA [49]. Methodologically speaking, most studies are association studies (case/control and cohort type), and two approaches have been done. In the most common approach (which for purposes of this chapter section are going to be called specific SNP association studies), the frequency of one or more known SNPs present in genes coding defined molecular candidates involved in the pro- or anti-inflammatory responses (e.g., alpha tumoral necrosis factor gene) is compared between a specific phenotypically defined interest group (patients with a confirmed specific infectious scenario as sepsis or IE) and a control group, usually consisting of a group of healthy blood donors ideally with an ethnicity equal to the interest group. If there are statistically significant differences in the frequency of the SNPs between groups, authors take this as proof that such genetic differences are implicated in the specific way that the study population responds to infection. The other approach is a type of study called genome-wide association studies (GWAS). As the previously described type of study, GWAS are association studies (most frequently case–control studies) but differ in that the frequency of most known SNPs is measured in the whole genome of the cases (infected group) and controls (healthy blood donors). When a statistically significant difference is found, authors take this as proof that such genetic variability is responsible for the difference in outcomes and then hypothesize, based in the location of the SNPs, about the biological plausibility of the association given the gene that is affected.

5.2 The evidence in sepsis

A large number of specific SNP association studies have been conducted respecting the most important effector molecules in response to sepsis and also some GWAS.

5.3 Tumor necrosis factor alpha

In response to an infectious stimuli, such as lipopolysaccharides (LPS), tumor necrosis factor α (TNF-α) is a cytokine that is released early mainly by macrophages, and it is a principal mediator of the inflammatory response to infection which stimulates acute inflammation by its action on different cells, such as endothelial cells and leukocytes [50].

Many studies have been done in an attempt to determine if specific SNPs in the TNF alpha factor gene are implicated in sepsis susceptibility with conflicting results. A recent meta-analysis from Zhang et al. [51] which included 23 articles that evaluated the effects of TNF-α rs1800629 and rs361525 polymorphisms on sepsis risk found that TNF-α rs1800629 was associated with increased sepsis risk in the overall population in four genetic models, including adenosine (A) vs. guanine (G) ($p < 0.001$, odds ratio (OR) = 1.32), GA vs. GG ($p < 0.001$, OR = 1.46), GA + AA vs. GG ($p < 0.001$, OR = 1.46), and carrier A vs. carrier G ($p < 0.001$, OR = 1.32). These results suggest an implication of these genetic variations with an increased susceptibility for sepsis development.

5.4 Tumor necrosis factor beta (TNF-β)

TNF-β is a cytokine produced by T lymphocytes similar to TNF-α and binds to TNF receptors. It activates endothelial cells and neutrophils and is a mediator of acute inflammatory response, providing a link between T-cell activation and inflammation. These effects are the same as those of TNF-α, consistent with their binding to the same receptors. However, as the quantity of TNF-β is much less than that of TNF-α made by lipopolysaccharide-stimulated mononuclear phagocytes, TNF-β is not readily detected in the circulation. For this reason, TNF-β is usually a local cytokine and not a mediator of systemic injury. A single nucleotide polymorphism has been found at position +252 in the first intron of the TNF-β gene and consists of a G in the wild-type allele (TNFB1) and an A in the variant allele (TNFB2). Known as the Nco1 polymorphism, it has been proposed as a potentially influential locus in many inflammatory conditions. Delongui et al. studied the association of the TNF-β Nco1 genetic polymorphism with susceptibility to sepsis in 60 patients diagnosed with sepsis and in 148 healthy blood donors. Among the septic patients, the allelic frequencies of TNFB1 and TNFB2 were 0.2833 and 0.7166, respectively, and they differed from those observed in the blood donors (p = 0.02). The TNFB2 allele frequency was higher in the septic patients than in the controls [OR = 1.65 (CI 95% 1.02–2.69), p = 0.0315], all this suggesting an implication in susceptibility to sepsis [52].

5.5 Interleukin 10 (IL-10)

IL-10 has beneficial anti-inflammatory properties; however, an excess of IL-10 has been reported to induce immunosuppression in bacterial sepsis. Published data demonstrates that lower production of IL-10 from stimulated peripheral blood mononuclear cells (PBMC) from septic patients is significantly correlated with favorable disease outcome [53]. Stanilova et al. [54] investigated the −1082 (A/G) polymorphism in the promoter of the IL-10 gene by measuring IL-10 production from stimulated peripheral blood mononuclear cells (PBMC) and to evaluate the relationship of this polymorphism with susceptibility to severe sepsis and its outcome. They found that carriage of at least one copy of IL-10-1082 G allele in sepsis patients and in healthy controls resulted in a statistically significant increase in IL-10 production from stimulated PBMC. Patients who survived sepsis had a significant decrease of IL-10-1082 allele G frequency, compared with controls (17 vs. 47.2%; p = 0.012). This suggests that this genetic variation has an impact in IL-10 production and in the outcomes of septic patients [55].

5.6 Interleukin-1 receptor antagonist gene (IL-1 Ra)

Interleukin 1β (IL-1β) is a potent pro-inflammatory cytokine implicated in the development of chronic inflammatory disorders. IL-1β signaling is blocked by IL-1 Ra, a natural regulator of IL-1 cytokines. IL-1 Ra binds to the IL-1 receptor and thereby prevents binding of both IL-1a and IL-1b [56]. F. Arnalich et al. aimed to determine the influence of the polymorphism within the intron 2 of the IL-1RNa (IL-RNa*) on the outcome of severe sepsis. A group of 78 patients with severe sepsis (51 survivors and 27 non-survivors) was compared with a healthy control group of 130 blood donors and 56 patients with uncomplicated pneumonia. They found a significant association between IL-1RN* polymorphism and survival. After adjusting for age and APACHE II score, they did a multiple logistic regression analysis that showed that patients' homozygotes for the allele *2 had 6·47 times more risk of death (95% CI 1·01–41·47, p = 0.04). These authors concluded that these genetic mutations might be implicated in an increased risk of death in septic patients [57].

5.7 High-mobility group box 1 protein (HMGB1)

HMGB1 is a pleiotropic cytokine that has been implicated in the pathophysiology of systemic inflammatory response syndrome (SIRS) and sepsis. HMGB1 is measurable in the systemic circulation in response to severe injury. This protein has the propensity to bind to a variety of inflammatory mediators such as lipopolysaccharide and pro-inflammatory cytokines, including IL-1. The role of HMGB1 as an endogenous molecule facilitates immune responses and has an important role in homeostasis between tissue and disease. HMGB1 is implicated in the pathophysiology of a variety of inflammatory diseases, and it has been found that variation in the HMGB1 gene is associated with mortality in patients with systemic inflammatory response syndrome [58]. Kornblit et al. performed a long-term, 4-year study comparing HMGB1 sequencing data in 239 intensive care unit (ICU) patients with HMGB1 blood levels and clinical outcomes. The promoter variant −1377delA was associated with a markedly reduced long-term survival rate after ICU admission in SIRS patients. There was also a significant interaction with a polymorphism within the coding region of the HMGB1 gene at position 982 (C > T) in exon 4; carriers had an increased frequency of early death from infection [59].

5.8 Toll-like receptor 2 (TLR2)

TLRs are a group of pattern recognition receptors. They play important roles in regulating inflammatory reactions and activating adaptive immune response to eliminate infective pathogens [60]. TLR2, a key member of TLR family, can recognize a variety of bacterial lipoproteins. The mechanism of TLR2-recognizing lipoproteins has been elucidated; after TLR2 recognizes lipoproteins, it activates MyD88 adaptor-like protein and initiates a signaling pathway, which induces further immune response [61]. This evidence puts TLR2 gene as an appealing candidate for determining sepsis risk. In a recent meta-analysis, Gao et al. [62] analyzed a total of 12 studies (11 records) with 898 cases and 1517 controls examined to determine the association between the TLR2 Arg753Gln polymorphism and sepsis risk. The combined results of the overall comparison indicated that there were significant associations between the TLR2 Arg753Gln polymorphism and sepsis risk under the allele comparison model and the dominant model, respectively (for A vs. G, OR 1.76, 95% CI 1.05–2.95, $p = 0.03$; for AA/GA vs. GG, OR 1.92, 95% CI 1.11–3.32, $p = 0.02$).

5.9 Genome-wide association study

Rautanen et al. [63] did a genome-wide association study in three independent cohorts of white adult patients admitted to ICU with sepsis, severe sepsis, or septic shock due to pneumonia or intra-abdominal infection ($n = 2534$ patients). The primary outcome was 28-day survival. Results for the three cohorts of patients with sepsis due to pneumonia were combined in a meta-analysis of 1553 patients. The most significantly associated SNPs were genotyped in a further 538 white patients with sepsis due to pneumonia (an independent fourth cohort), of whom 106 died. In the genome-wide meta-analysis of three independent pneumonia cohorts, common variants in the FER gene were strongly associated with survival ($p = 9{\cdot}7 \times 10–8$; OR 0·52 [95% CI 0·41–0·66]). Genotyping of the additional fourth cohort strengthened the evidence for association with survival ($p = 5{\cdot}6 \times 10–8$; OR 0·56 [0·45–0·69]).

5.10 The evidence in infective endocarditis

There are many risk factors described for the development of IE; nevertheless up to 30–50% of patients with this diagnosis does not have any known risk factor [64]. Therefore, as in sepsis per se, there is thought to be immunogenetic influences that affect the risk of development and outcomes in IE. However, in comparison to sepsis, evidence of the immunogenetic influence on the susceptibility and outcomes of IE is less robust. Golovkin et al. [65] hypothesized that inherited variation in TLR and triggering receptor expressed on myeloid cells (TREMs) genes may affect individual susceptibility to IE. They conducted a specific SNP study in which the distribution of genotypes and alleles of the TLR1, TLR2, TLR4, TLR6, and TREM-1 gene polymorphisms was investigated in 110 Caucasian subjects with IE and 300 matched healthy blood donors. ORs with 95% CI were calculated. They found that C/C genotype of the rs3775073 polymorphism within TLR6 gene was associated with a decreased risk of IE (OR = 0.51, 95% CI = 0.26–0.97, p = 0.032) according to the recessive model; however, there was no association between the other investigated SNPs within TLR andTREM-1 genes and IE.

Moreau et al. [66] conducted a GWAS of 67 patients with definite native valve *S. aureus* IE (cases) and 72 matched native valve patients with *S. aureus* bacteremia but without IE (controls). Unfortunately, no SNPs were significantly associated with *S. aureus* IE at the genome-wide level ($p < 5 \times 10^{-8}$). Four suggestive SNPs ($p < 0.00001$) were located on one locus on chromosome 3, near the genes CLDN11 and SLC7A14. For all, the frequency of the minor allele was lower in cases than in controls, suggesting a protective effect against *S. aureus* IE. The same association was observed using an independent Danish verification cohort of *Staphylococcus aureus* bacteremia with (n = 57) and without (n = 123) IE. An ex vivo analysis of aortic valve tissues revealed that *S. aureus* IE associated SNPs mentioned above were associated with significantly higher mRNA expression levels of SLC7A14, which is a cationic amino acid transporter protein. These results suggest an IE-protective effect of SNPs on chromosome 3 during *S. aureus* bacteremia. The authors concluded that the effects of protective minor alleles may be mediated by increasing expression levels of SLC7A14 in valve tissues.

6. Inflammation and oxidative stress

The modern mitochondria have an evolution of more than a billion years, originating as an invading *Eubacterium* in early eukaryotic cells. The knowledge of the structure, functionality, and the similarities of the DNA between mitochondria and bacteria strongly prove the endosymbiotic origin of the mitochondria. Of the 1000 or more mitochondrial proteins, only 13 are encoded by the mitochondrial genome, the rest is transcribed and translated into the nuclear genome and transported to the inner mitochondrial membrane [67].

In the heart the populations of mitochondria include subsarcolemmal mitochondria, which are more susceptible to injury. Subsarcolemmal mitochondria provide energy for membrane-related processes, including signal transduction, ion exchange, and substrate transport, whereas the intermyofibrillar mitochondria more directly support muscle contraction [68].

The mitochondrial oxidative phosphorylation process is responsible for the conversion of macronutrient energy (e.g., glucose, fatty acids, and amino acids) into ATP through a set of coordinated and highly coupled reactions where the macronutrients are oxidized and the oxygen is reduced to water and adenosine diphosphate (ADP) is phosphorylated to ATP.

6.1 Chemiosmotic hypothesis

In the chemiosmotic hypothesis [69], the proton gradient is formed by removing H^+ from the interior (matrix), while the negative charges remain inside, largely as OH^- ions; the pH on the outer face of the membrane (intermembrane space) can reach a pH of 5.5, while the pH just at the inner side (matrix) of the same can reach 8.5; this gradient is 3 pH units. Recall that the pH is equal to - log. of $[H^+]$, and therefore 3 units of pH mean that the $\Delta H^+ = 1000$ between both faces of the membrane, that is to say there are 1000 times more H^+ in the intermembrane space than on the side of the membrane that is in contact with the mitochondrial matrix (**Figure 1**).

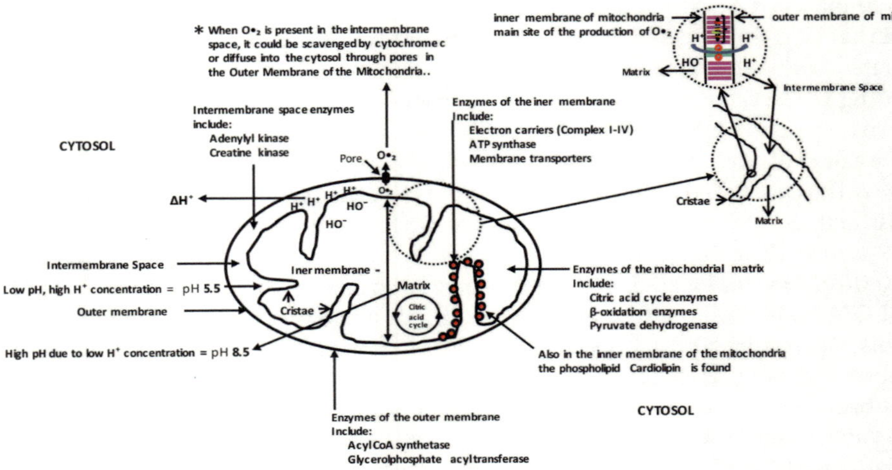

Figure 1.
The creation of a proton gradient (ΔH^+) in the intermembrane space is produced by the chain of electron transport and the synthesis of ATP synthase, which is maintained by the electrons that pass from the reducing equivalents (NADH, FADH2) to the cytochromes along the inner membrane of the mitochondria. ATP synthase uses that gradient to generate ATP. The two processes are associated with the inner membrane of the mitochondria in the mitochondrial crests. Note that the enzymes of the citric acid cycle and β-oxidation are contained in mitochondria, together with the respiratory chain, which collects and transports reducing equivalents, directing them to their final reaction with oxygen to form water, and the machinery for oxidative phosphorylation, the process by which the liberated free energy is trapped as high-energy phosphate. Source: Botham and Mayes [70].

The process begins when carbon substrates enter the tricarboxylic acid cycle through acetyl CoA or anaplerotic reactions. Oxidation of these substrates generates reducing equivalents in the form of NADH and FADH2, which provide electron fluxes through the complexes of the respiratory chain, complex I (NADH dehydrogenase) and complex II (succinate dehydrogenase). The flow of electrons through complexes I and II converges in complex III (ubiquinone-cytochrome c reductase), together with electrons from electron transfer flavoproteins (beta oxidation), although the mobile electron carrier coenzyme Q as second mobile electron carrier transfers electrons to the IV complex (cytochrome c oxidase) where they are finally transferred to oxygen, producing water. A gradient of protons (an electrochemical gradient) through the inner mitochondrial membrane is generated by the action of electron transport through complexes I, III, and IV. The potential energy of this gradient is exploited by the V (ATP synthase) complex to phosphorylate ADP to ATP [71]. It is clear that the maintenance of the mitochondrial membrane potential through the transport of electrons is critical for the proper function of the organelle and, therefore, of the cell and of ascending form of organs and systems.

6.2 Reactive oxygen species

In the process of mitochondrial respiration, the generation of reactive oxygen species (ROS) is generally a cascade of reactions that begins with the production of superoxide $O{\bullet}_2$. The oxidative stress is defined as an imbalance that favors ROS production on antioxidant defenses; most ROS are products of mitochondrial respiration. Approximately 1–2% of the molecular oxygen consumed during the process of mitochondria respiration is converted to superoxide radicals. Briefly, the reduction of an electron of molecular oxygen produces a relatively stable intermediate, the superoxide anion ($O{\bullet}_2$); the importance of this is that it serves as the precursor to most ROS.

Therefore, it is very important to take into account the sources that generate it. There is evidence that most of the $O{\bullet}_2$ generated by intact mammalian mitochondria in vitro is produced by complex I. The production of superoxide—$O{\bullet}_2$—is mainly carried out in the inner mitochondrial membrane (IMM) together with complex III [72, 73]. On the other hand, the production of $O{\bullet}_2$ is stimulated by the presence of succinate (substrate of complex II) [74]. Ubiquinone as part of the respiratory chain binds complexes I with II and II with III which is also important for the formation of $O{\bullet}_2$ by complex III [75]. Oxidation of ubiquinone—Q cycle—and unstable semiquinone also generates $O{\bullet}_2$ (**Figure 2**).

The Q cycle couples electron transfer to proton transport in complex III electrons are passed from QH_2 to cytochrome c via complex III (Q-cytochrome c oxidoreductase) as described in **Figure 2**.

$$QH_2 + 2\text{cyt } c_{\text{oxidized}} + 2H^+ \text{ matrix} \quad (1)$$

$$Q + 2\text{cyt } c_{\text{reduced}} + 4H^+ \text{ intermembrane space} \quad (2)$$

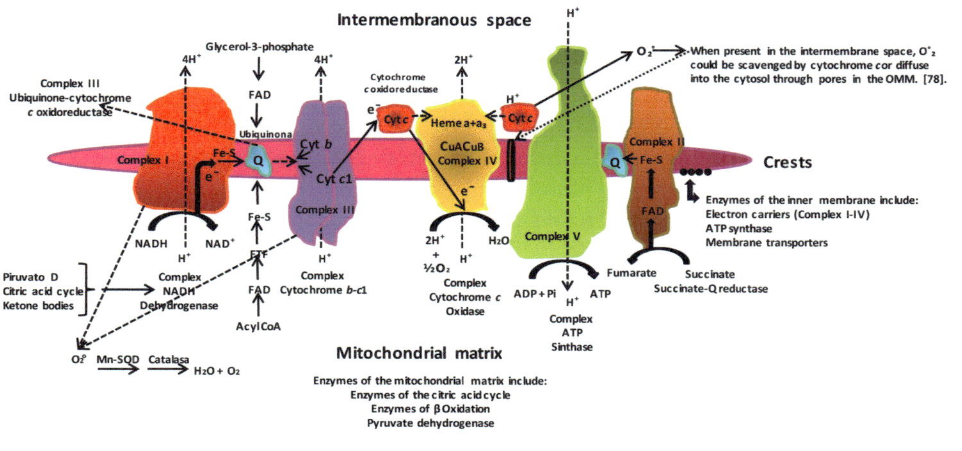

Figure 2.
The flavin adenine dinucleotide (FAD) can be reduced in reactions involving the transfer of two electrons (to form $FMNH_2$ or $FADH_2$), but they can also accept one electron to form the semi Quinone. Electron-transferring flavoprotein (ETF). Fe-S, iron–sulfur proteins (nonheme iron proteins). The Fe-S take part in single-electron transfer reactions in which one Fe atom undergoes oxidoreduction between Fe^{2+} and Fe^{3+}. Coenzyme Q (Q) (also called ubiquinone) (complex I). Cytochrome c, Q-cytochrome c oxidoreductase (complex III), which passes the electrons on to cytochrome c; and cytochrome c oxidase (complex IV), which completes the chain, passing the electrons to O_2 and causing it to be reduced to H_2O. Q and cytochrome c are mobile. Q diffuses rapidly within the membrane, while cytochrome c is a soluble protein. Mn-SOD, manganese superoxide dismutase.

Superoxide rapidly dismutates into hydrogen peroxide spontaneously or at a low pH is catalyzed by superoxide dismutase. Other elements in the cascade of ROS generation are small molecules derived from oxygen, like the following: hydroxyl (OH•), peroxyl ($RO•_2$), and alkoxyl (RO•) and certain non-radicals that are oxidizing agents and/or are easily converted to radicals, such as hypochlorous acid (HOCl), ozone (O_3), singlet oxygen (½O_2), and hydrogen peroxide (H_2O_2). Nitrogen-containing oxidants, such as nitric oxide (NO), are called reactive nitrogen species (RNS), and the Fenton reaction catalyzed by iron leads to the generation of hydroxyl radical [76, 77]. The dismutation of superoxide anions by superoxide dismutases results in the production of H_2O_2. The mitochondria contribute 20–30% of the stable cytosolic concentration of H_2O_2 [78]; the subsequent interaction of H_2O_2 and $O•_2$ in a Haber-Weiss reaction, or the cleavage of H_2O_2 driven by Fe^{2+}- (or Cu^{2+}), can generate the highly reactive hydroxyl radical (OH•).

The Haber-Weiss reaction [79] may occur as a consequence of oxidative stress. The reaction is catalyzed by the iron in oxidation state (III); the first step of the catalytic cycle is produced by the reduction of the ferric cation to ferrous cation:

$$Fe_3{}^{+} + •O^{-}{}_2 \rightarrow Fe_2{}^{+} + O_2 \quad (3)$$

The second step is a reaction from Fenton:

$$Fe^{2+} + H_2O_2 \rightarrow Fe^{3+} + OH^{-} + •OH \quad (4)$$

6.3 Superoxide dismutases

Briefly, superoxide dismutases (SOD) are a group of metalloenzymes (containing Fe, Mn, or Cu and Zn) that catalyze the disproportionation of superoxide free radical (2O•) to form hydrogen peroxide and oxygen as shown below:

$$2•O_2 + 2H^{+} \Leftrightarrow H_2O_2 + O_2 \quad (5)$$

In some cell types, CuZnSOD is present in the mitochondrial intermembrane space, where it can convert $O•_2$ to H_2O_2, thus permitting further diffusion into the cytosol.

Superoxide rapidly dismutates into hydrogen peroxide spontaneously or at a low pH is catalyzed by sequential actions of superoxide dismutase (SOD), and catalase converts superoxide into oxygen and water. Other elements in the cascade of ROS generation are small molecules derived from oxygen, which also include oxygen radicals [80].

Because ROS are biologically damaging, they need to be metabolized to prevent the damage they can cause when interacting with other compounds, for which the cell counts with mechanisms that avoid it like SOD. However, when the formation of ROS increases, they have the capacity to deteriorate mitochondrial function and jeopardize cell survival in different ways, where the mitochondrion seems to be responsible for regulating apoptosis [81]. ROS are a major threat to encode, transfer, and transport electrons and generate ATP by directly damaging mitochondrial DNA (mtDNA) which encodes 13 polypeptides, 12 transfer RNAs (tRNAs), and 2 ribosomal RNAs (rRNAs). All of them are essential in the chain of transport of electrons for the production of ATP, so when interacting with them, oxidative phosphorylation and therefore energy genesis is compromised [67]. ROS, and the release of proapoptotic proteins from the intermembrane space of mitochondria, triggers the activation of cell death.

7. Nicotinamide adenine dinucleotide phosphate oxidase

7.1 NADPH oxidase

The heart has the highest oxygen uptake rate in the human body, and the oxygen consumption is normally 8–13 mL 100 g^{-1} min^{-1} at rest [82]. The cellular sources in the genesis of ROS in the heart include cardiac myocytes, endothelial cells, and neutrophils. Within cardiac myocytes, ROS can be produced by several mechanisms, including the transport of mitochondrial electrons, NADPH oxidase (nicotinamide adenine dinucleotide phosphate oxidase), and xanthine dehydrogenase/xanthine oxidase. To meet the high demand for ATP synthesis, cardiac myocytes therefore have the highest volume density of mitochondria in the entire human body.

NADPH oxidase with its isoforms generically called NOX is the major source of ROS (reactive oxygen species) in biological systems. NOX proteins are involved in a plethora of pathophysiological conditions, so it is important to note that the functions of NOX proteins in different tissues are influenced by the activity of other oxidases and peroxidases, such as myeloperoxidase, xanthine oxidase, and hemoxygenase [83].

In the heart, the cardiomyocyte NADPH oxidase seems to be the main source of production of ROS from the heart in failure [84, 85].

NADPH oxidases are present in phagocytes and in a wide variety of non-phagocytic cells. NADPH generates superoxide by transferring electrons from NADPH into the cell through the membrane and coupling them to molecular oxygen to produce superoxide anion. Structurally, NADPH oxidase is an enzyme that has several components: it includes two integral membrane proteins, the glycoprotein gp. 1 Phox and the adapter protein p22 (phox), which together form the heterodimeric b558 flavocytochrome that form the nucleus of the enzyme. During the resting state, the multidomain regulatory subunits p40P (phox), p47 (phox), and p67 (Phox) are located in the cytosol organized as a complex. Activation of phagocytic NADPH oxidase occurs through a complex series of protein interactions.

The products that activate it are angiotensin II, endothelin-1, TNF-α, and mechanical forces. The cardiomyocyte NADPH oxidase and any other NADPH oxidase when stimulated generates large amounts of ($O•_2$), which dismutes to H_2O_2; both in the tissue presence of iron and H_2O_2, increase the production of ROS, lead to the production of the HO• radical; these are highly reactive and can induce peroxidative damage of molecules within reach such as lipids, proteins, carbohydrates, nucleic acids, and membranes, resulting in the increase of reactive substances thiobarbituric acid (TBARS) in patients with heart failure.

This suggests that some pro-inflammatory products can activate a pathway to generate oxidative stress damage through the NADPH oxidase and increase the biological damage to the heart by ROS which correlates with left ventricular dysfunction [86]. Even more, the fact that NADPH oxidase is activated by pro-inflammatory products suggests a link with the genesis of oxidative stress.

Of the infectious processes in the heart on the balance of oxidants and antioxidants in the myocardium little is known. IE in which heart valves are usually affected, generating refractory congestive heart failure, is accompanied by a very important inflammatory response, both local and systemic with high circulating concentrations of IL-6, IL-2R, and IL-1β [87]. In the case of infective endocarditis, the interaction of the infectious agent and its products (chemotactic, formylated, and lipopolysaccharide peptides) with monocytes and polymorphonuclear cells can increase the production of ROS through the activation of NADPH oxidase, secondary to the inflammatory state.

IE induces an increase of pro-inflammatory cytokines, being able to stimulate ROS production in the myocardium and peroxidative damage to several molecules. The substances reactive to thiobarbituric acid (TBAR), in a study comparing cardiac tissue from patients with IE and patients with valvular heart disease (VHD) of rheumatic etiology; TBARs were increased 10 times more in IE than their controls with VHD [88].

8. Inducible nitric oxide synthase

In sepsis, endotoxins and cytokines stimulate the expression of inducible nitric oxide synthase (iNOS) and the overproduction of nitric oxide (NO) in various tissues; it also stimulates the excessive activity of NADPH oxidase that facilitates the expression of iNOS to produce large amounts of NO. The NADPH oxidases derived from ROS by activating the Jak2-IRF1 and JNK-AP1 pathways are necessary for the induction of iNOS. The main mechanism that regulates the activity of iNOS is the modulation of the transcription of the iNOS gene. The NO derived from iNOS and its metabolite peroxynitrite can contribute to the pathological alterations observed in sepsis, such as endothelial dysfunction, hypotension, and multiple organ failure [89].

The peroxynitrite anion $ONOO^-$

$$H_2O_2 + NO_2^- \rightarrow ONOO^- + H_2O \tag{6}$$

$$\bullet O_2^- + \bullet NO \rightarrow ONO_2^- \tag{7}$$

9. Metabolome and proteome

The composition of metabolites such as amino acids, intermediate products of the Krebs cycle, and acylcarnitines (metabolome) and protein complement expressed in cells, tissues, or body fluids (proteome) of survivors of sepsis and non-survivors was analyzed in patients who studied with sepsis by three different pathogens, *S. pneumoniae*, *S. aureus*, or *E. coli*. The main differences between survivors and non-survivors were those highlighted in their metabolome and proteome. For example, nine proteins involved in the transport of fatty acids were decreased in non-survivors of sepsis, suggesting a defect in β-oxidation. The nonacceptance and nonuse of fatty acids by the mitochondria led to an accumulation of acylcarnitines in the plasma; another predictive marker is that glycolysis and gluconeogenesis were also markedly different. Survivors of sepsis showed decreased levels of citrate, malate, glycerol, glycerol 3-phosphate, phosphate, and glucogenic and ketogenic amino acids, while non-survivors showed elevated levels of citrate, malate, pyruvate, dihydroxyacetone, lactate, phosphate, and gluconeogenic amino acids [90]. That is to say that the pathways for the transport of fatty acids, as well as glycolysis and gluconeogenesis, are damaged, so the substrate is low, and they are not used by the mitochondria.

10. Acetylome

Acetylome analysis identified a subpopulation of mitochondrial proteins that was sensitive to changes in the NADH/NAD+ ratio. Hyperacetylation induced by mitochondrial dysfunction is a positive regulator of pathological remodeling in the heart of mice with *primary or acquired* mitochondrial dysfunction, as well as in humans with heart failure. Hyperacetylation of mitochondrial malate–aspartate shuttle (MAS) proteins impaired the transport and oxidation of cytosolic NADH in the mitochondria, resulting in altered cytosolic redox state and energy deficiency. Furthermore, acetylation of oligomycin-sensitive conferring protein at lysine-70 in adenosine triphosphate synthase complex promoted its interaction with cyclophilin D and sensitized the opening of mitochondrial permeability transition pore. There are two different mechanisms that point to the proteins of hyperacetylation, i.e., MAS and the regulators of mitochondrial permeability transition pore (mPTP), which mediate an increase in heart failure. Both could be fixed by normalizing the NAD+ redox balance either genetically or pharmacologically [91].

11. *Q* and cytochrome *c*

Q and cytochrome *c* (Cyt*c*) are mobile. *Q* diffuses rapidly within the membrane, while cytochrome *c* is a soluble protein that contains a peptide sequence located at the C-terminus of the protein [92] that allows it to cross the cell membranes in a nontraditional way. This property of Cyt*c* was used in a study in mice, which were subject to ligation and cecal puncture; they underwent sepsis and damage to mitochondrial respiration, which was restored with the injection i.v. of Cyt*c* [93]. The treatment led to an uptake of Cyt*c* into the cardiomyocytes, and survival increased from 15% for the sepsis control group to about 50% in mice that were also injected with Cytc [94].

12. Deregulated apoptosis and multiple organ failure

The death of cells of the immune system by deregulated apoptosis contributes to the dysfunction of the immune system and multiple organ failure (MOF) which is observed in sepsis. The immune cells most affected by this dysregulated apoptotic cell death appear to be lymphocytes [95]. Extensive lymphocytic apoptosis mediated by caspase-3 in sepsis may contribute to impaired immune response in septic patients [96]. Lymphocyte loss occurs by both death receptor and mitochondrial-mediated apoptosis, suggesting that there may be multiple triggers for lymphocyte apoptosis [97, 98].

Apoptosis in the immune system is a pathological event in sepsis which has been considered a therapeutic goal. Studies on sepsis in experimental animals suggest that the loss of lymphocytes during sepsis may be due to deregulated apoptosis and that it appears to be secondary to a variety of mediators that carry out both "intrinsic" and "extrinsic" cell death pathways.

In experimental animals, lymphocyte apoptosis is frequently seen 12 h after the onset of experimental polymicrobial sepsis in the thymus, spleen, and lymphoid tissues associated with the intestine. It has been suggested that deregulated lymphocytic apoptosis results in reduced septic survival through loss of lymphocytes, resulting in multiple organ failure and ultimately death. Lymphocyte apoptosis in the thymus appears to occur 4 h after the onset of sepsis and is independent of the effects of endotoxin or death receptors. Apoptosis in the spleen appears to be particularly important in mortality from sepsis, by an increase of the splenic apoptosis of lymphocytes in experimental animals after the cecal ligation and puncture (CLP) which results in a reduced survival [99].

In septic humans apoptosis does not seem to be generalized, since in these patients only extensive lymphocytic apoptosis was demonstrated, which suggests a damaged immune response, suggesting that other mechanisms apart from cell death participate in the conditions associated with mortality [100]. For example, hyperglycemia induces the expression of leukocyte adhesion molecules, such as the intercellular adhesion molecule (ICAM) and vascular cell adhesion molecule (VCAM), which is suppressed by treatment with insulin. Another example is the impairment induced by hyperglycemia in the function of neutrophils, including chemotaxis, phagocytosis, and respiratory function, which is attenuated with insulin [101].

13. Conclusions

As we observed, the epidemiology of IE has changed over time. *S. aureus* is currently the most important pathological agent as a cause of IE [4, 102]. The age group with greater participation is the older adult due to their comorbidities, especially cardiac ones, with the need for valve prosthesis placement, and vascular approach for the placement of cardiac pacemakers.

The existence of an immunogenetic influence in the risk and outcomes of infectious diseases has been well stablished. In the cases of IE and sepsis, investigation is ongoing to clearly define the specific genetic anomalies that contribute to this influence. The study of SNPs has been a good start in the understanding of the phenomena; nevertheless at the light of the information derived from their study, they do not seem sufficient to explain the whole participation of genetics in the sepsis and IE equation. Other types of genetic abnormalities might also participate, and it might be worth exploring [103]. Even though there is a large body of studies with positive results, there are also lots of contradictory and conflicting findings that make it difficult to make definitive conclusions. Even more, according to a systematic review made to determine the methodological quality of SNP association studies with sepsis, most of the studies could improve a lot methodologically speaking in terms of control group selection, genetic assay technique, study blinding, statistical interpretation, study replication, study size, and power.

Finally, the sequence of events that begin with an infectious state, such as IE, alerts and promotes inflammation through the immune system, both cellular and humoral to eliminate the infectious agent; however, this has the ability to evade the immune system.

In its evolution, the germ also generated the possibility of survival through the acquisition of resistance to external agents, such as antibiotics, which can perpetuate the septic process, increasing the production of reactive O_2 species both locally (cell-mitochondria) and systemic level (neutrophil-monocytes-macrophage-endothelium) together with the products that generate the interaction infectious agent-immune system.

The activity of antioxidant enzymes is exceeded, so that ROS cannot be eliminated, generating a state of oxidative stress, with a profound effect on the mitochondrial level by breaking the chain of electron transport, and, consequently, the genesis of the energy is compromised.

The repercussion of this sequence of events, both at the cardiac level and at the systemic level, is manifested by the failure of one or several organs.

In a schematic way, the sequence of events of a patient with IE who has a severe evolution and finally dies of multiple organ failure is shown (**Figure 3**).

Different studies explore areas of compromise such as metabolome and proteome in which it is observed that glycolysis, gluconeogenesis, and fatty acid

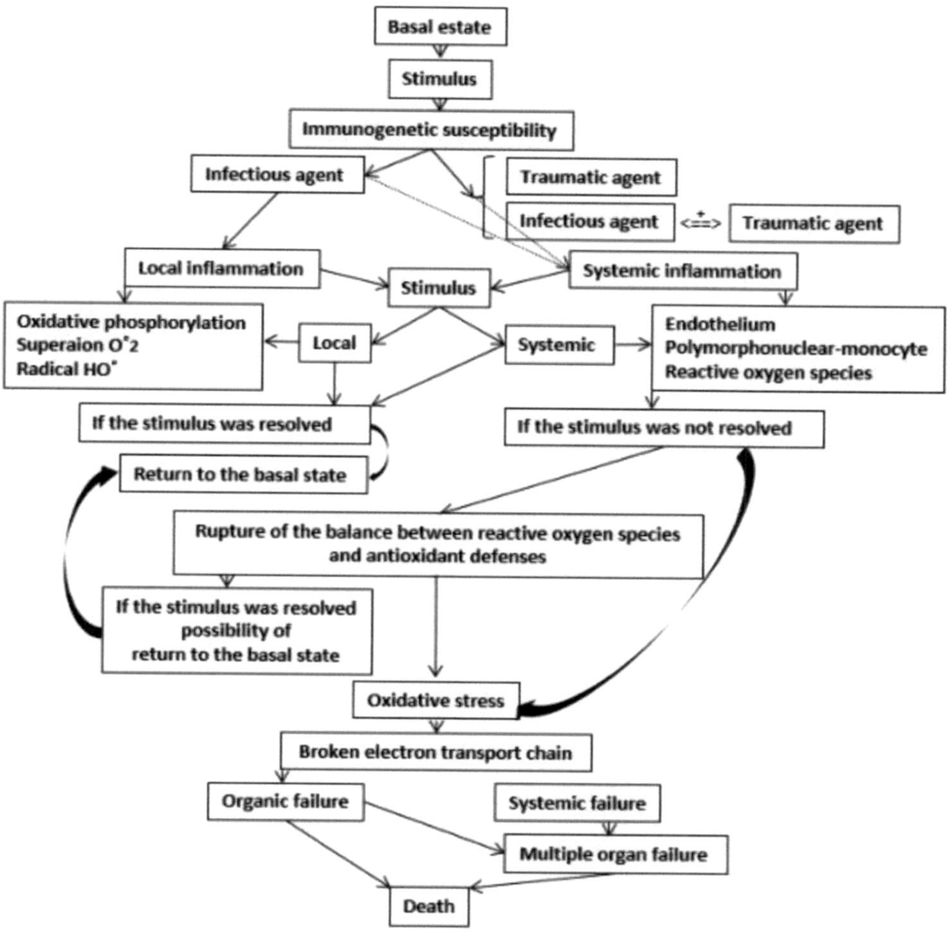

Figure 3.
Schematic representation of the sequence of events of a patient with IE who has a severe evolution and finally dies of multiple organ failure.

transport are damaged, so the substrate is low and the few substrates are not used by the mitochondria, which generates attention in processes to be repaired.

In another (acetylome) the possibility of normalizing the NAD + redox balance is observed both genetically and pharmacologically in the treatment of heart failure [91].

The observations of the behavior of cytochrome c, being a mobile complex molecule and crossing cell membranes, made it possible for cytochrome c to enter into cardiomyocytes to improve mitochondrial respiration, improving the survival of septic mice [92–94]. This open a very attractive opportunity in the treatment of septic patients with heart failure as in IE when in the future we use complex molecules, i.v., in the treatment of these patients.

There are still many areas in which it is necessary to continue researching in the clinical area as well as in the bacteriological, biochemical, and biomolecular areas in addition to other types of tools to observe systemic inflammation, through mathematical modulation and systems-based models of inflammation [104, 105], and the severity of a septic patient due to the complexity of losing the cardiac bioelectrical signal and how it recovers the complexity if the patient survives the septic event have also been considered [106].

Acknowledgements

Vet. Laura Yavarik Alvarado Avila. Faculty of Veterinary Medicine. National Autonomous University of Mexico UNAM, Mexico City, Mexico. We appreciate the support in the corrections and spelling suggestions made in this chapter on Infective Endocarditis.

Conflict of interest

None.

Acronyms and abbreviations

MRSA	methicillin-resistant *Staphylococcus aureus*
HssRS	hem sensor system
hrtAB	hem regulator transporter
bNOS	nitric oxide synthase hemoprotein
TNF	tumor necrosis factor alpha
IL	interleukin
HMGB1	high-mobility group box 1 protein
GRO alpha	growth-regulated oncogene
RANTES	regulated upon activation, normal T-cell expressed, and secreted
EE	endocardial endothelium
Et-1	endothelin-1
ON	nitric oxide
PG	prostaglandins
VEGF	vascular endothelial growth factor
SNP	single-nucleotide polymorphism
GWAS	genome-wide association studies
LPS	lipopolysaccharides
A	adenosine
G	guanine
PBMC	peripheral blood mononuclear cells
IL-RNa*	The interleukin 1receptor antagonist gene
APACHE II score	acute physiology and chronic health evaluation
SIRS	systemic inflammatory response syndrome
ICU	intensive care unit
TLR	toll-like receptor
MyD88	adaptor-like protein
FER gene	tyrosine-protein kinase
TREMs	triggering receptor expressed on myeloid cells
ADP	adenosine diphosphate
NADH	nicotinamide adenine dinucleotide phosphate
FADH	flavin adenine dinucleotide
ROS	reactive oxygen species
IMM	inner mitochondrial membrane
OH•	hydroxyl
$RO•_2$	peroxyl
RO•	alkoxyl

HOCl	hypochlorous acid
O_3	ozone
½O_2	singlet oxygen
H_2O_2	hydrogen peroxide
RNS	reactive nitrogen species
SOD	superoxide dismutases
2O•$_2$	superoxide free radical
CuZnSOD	copper, zinc-superoxide dismutase
mtDNA	mitochondrial DNA
tRNAs	transfer RNAs
rRNAs	ribosomal RNAs
NOX	NADPH oxidase generically called
phox	adapter protein p22
TBARS	reactive substances thiobarbituric acid
iNOS	inducible nitric oxide synthase
NO	nitric oxide
JNK-AP1	Jak2-IRF1 pathway genes (*IFNGR1, IFNGR2, JAK1, JAK2, STAT1, IRF1*)
MOF	multiple organ failure
MODS	multi-organ dysfunction syndrome
CLP	cecal ligation and puncture
ICAM	intercellular adhesion molecule
VCAM	vascular cell adhesion molecule

Author details

Pedro Eduardo Alvarado Rubio MD[1*], Roberto Brugada Molina MD[1], Pedro Eduardo Alvarado Ávila MD[2,3], Alejandro González Mora MD[1] and Cesar Augusto González López MD[1]

1 Institute of Security and Social Services for Workers of the state ISSSTE, Hospital Regional Lic. Adolfo López Mateos, Critical Care Unit, Mexico City, Mexico

2 National Institute of Medical Sciences and Nutrition Salvador Zubiran, Mexico

3 National Autonomous University of Mexico UNAM, Mexico City, Mexico

*Address all correspondence to: pancreatitis2@gmail.com

References

[1] Holland T et al. Infective endocarditis. Nature Reviews. Disease Primers. 2016;**2**:16059

[2] Wang A et al. Management considerations in infective endocarditis: A review. Journal of the American Medical Association. 2018;**320**:72-83. DOI: 10.1001/jama.2018.7596

[3] Cresti A et al. Epidemiological and mortality trends in infective endocarditis, a 17-year population-based prospective study. Cardiovascular Diagnosis and Therapy. 2017;7:27-35

[4] Slipczuk L, Codolosa JN, Davila CD, et al. Infective endocarditis epidemiology over five decades: A systematic review. PLoS One. 2013; **8**(12):e82665. DOI: 10.1371/journal.pone.0082665

[5] Baddour L et al. Infective endocarditis in adults. Diagnosis, antimicrobial therapy and management of complications. Circulation. 2015;**132**: 1435-1486

[6] Keynan Y et al. Infective endocarditis in the intensive care unit. Critical Care Clinics. 29 Oct 2013;**29**(4):923-951. DOI: 10.1016/j.ccc.2013.06.011. Epub 2013 Aug 17. Review. PMID: 24094385

[7] Bone RC et al. Definitions for sepsis and organ failure and guidelines for the use of innovative therapies in sepsis. The ACCP/SCCM Consensus Conference Committee. American College of Chest Physicians/Society of Critical Care Medicine. Chest. 1992;**101**: 1644-1655

[8] Levy M et al. 2001 SCCM/ESICM/ACCP/ATS/SIS international sepsis definitions conference. Critical Care Medicine. 2003;**31**:1250-1256

[9] Singer M et al. The third international definitions for sepsis and septic shock (sepsis 3). Journal of the American Medical Association. 2016; **315**:801-810

[10] Seymour C et al. Assessment of clinical criteria for sepsis for the third international consensus definitions for sepsis and septic shock (sepsis 3). Journal of the American Medical Association. 2016;**315**:762-774

[11] Cahill TJ, Prendergast BD. Infective endocarditis. Lancet. 2016;**387**: 882-893. DOI: 10.1016/S0140-6736(15)00067-7

[12] Krajinovic V et al. Association between cardiac surgery and mortality among patients with infective endocarditis complicated by sepsis and septic shock. Shock. 2018;**49**: 536-542

[13] Olmos C et al. Contemporary epidemiology and prognosis of septic shock in infective endocarditis. European Heart Journal. 2013;**34**: 1999-2006

[14] Wang A. The changing epidemiology of infective endocarditis. Journal of the American College of Cardiology May. 2012;**59**(22):1977-1978. DOI: 10.1016/j.jacc.2012.02.030

[15] Fleischauer AT, Ruhl L, Rhea S, Barnes E. Hospitalizations for endocarditis and associated health care costs among persons with diagnosed drug dependence—North Carolina, 2010–2015. Morbidity and Mortality Weekly Report. 2017;**66**(22): 569-573. DOI: 10.15585/mmwr.mm6622a1

[16] Bor DH et al. Infective endocarditis in the U.S., 1998–2009: A nationwide study. PLoS One. 2013;**8**:e60033

[17] Rangel F et al. Natural history of the systemic inflammatory response syndrome (SIRS). A prospective study. Journal of the American Medical Association. 1995;**273**:117-123

[18] Barbara E et al. Internalization of *Staphylococcus aureus* by endothelial cells induces apoptosis. Infection and Immunity. 1998;**66**:5994-5998

[19] Lowy FD, Fant J, Higgins LL, Ogawa SK, Hatcher VB. *Staphylococcus aureus*—Human endothelial cell interactions. Journal of Ultrastructure and Molecular Structure Research. 1988;**98**:137-146

[20] Hamill RJ, Vann JM, Proctor RA. Phagocytosis of *Staphylococcus aureus* by cultured bovine endothelial cells: Model for postadherence events in endovascular infections. Infection and Immunity. 1986;**54**:833-836

[21] Ogawa SK, Yurberg ER, Hatcher VB, Levitt MA, Lowy FD. Bacterial adherence to human endothelial cells in vitro. Infection and Immunity. 1985; **50**:218-224

[22] Hammer ND, Reniere ML, Cassat JE, Zhang Y, Hirsch AO, Indriati Hood M, et al. Two heme-dependent terminal oxidases power *Staphylococcus aureus* organ-specific colonization of the vertebrate host. mBio Journal. 2013;**4**: e00241

[23] Skaar EP, Humayun M, Bae T, DeBord KL, Schneewind O. Iron-source preference of *Staphylococcus aureus* infections. Science. 2004;**305**:1626-1628

[24] Torres VJ, Pishchany G, Humayun M, Schneewind O, Skaar EP. *Staphylococcus aureus* IsdB is a hemoglobin receptor required for heme iron utilization. Journal of Bacteriology. 2006;**188**:8421-8429

[25] Kuechenmeister L, Dunman PM, Skaar EP. *Staphylococcus aureus* HrtA is an ATPase required for protection against heme toxicity and prevention of a transcriptional heme stress response. Journal of Bacteriology. 2008;**190**: 3588-3596

[26] Matthew C et al. Bacterial nitric oxide synthase is required for the *Staphylococcus aureus* response to heme stress. ACS Infectious Diseases. 2016;**2**: 572-578

[27] McNicholas S. Cytokine responses to *Staphylococcus aureus* bloodstream infection differ between patient cohorts that have different clinical courses of infection. Infectious Diseases. 2014;**14**: 580

[28] Barrett FF, Gehee M, Jr RF, Finland M. Methicillin-resistant *Staphylococcus aureus* at Boston City Hospital. Bacteriologic and epidemiologic observations. The New England Journal of Medicine. 1968;**279**:441-448

[29] Klevens RM, Edwards JR, Tenover FC, McDonald LC, Horan T, Gaynes R, et al. Changes in the epidemiology of methicillin resistant *Staphylococcus aureus* in intensive care units in US hospitals, 1992–2003. Clinical Infectious Diseases. 2006;**42**:389-391

[30] Wisplinghoff H, Bischoff T, Tallent SM, Seifert H, Wenzel RP, Edmond MB. Nosocomial bloodstream infections in US hospitals: Analysis of 24,179 cases from prospective nationwide surveillance study. Clinical Infectious Diseases. 2004;**39**:309-317

[31] Friedman N et al. Health care-associated bloodstream infections in adults: A reason to change the accepted definition of community-acquired infections. Annals of Internal Medicine. 2002;**137**:791-797

[32] Kock R, Becker K, Cookson B, van Gemert-Pijnen JE, Harbarth S, Kluytmans J, et al. Methicillin-resistant

Staphylococcus aureus (MRSA): Burden of disease and control challenges in Europe. Euro Surveillance. 2010;**15**: 19688

[33] Brutsaert DL. Cardiac endothelial-myocardial signaling: It's role in cardiac growth, contractile performance, and rhythmicity. Physiological Reviews. 2003;**83**:59-115

[34] Mohananey D et al. Association of the size of vegetation with embolic risk in patients with infectious endocarditis: A systematic review and meta-analysis. JAMA Internal Medicine. 2018;**178**: 502-510

[35] Cardullo AC, Silvers DN, Grossman ME. Janeway lesions and Osler's nodes: A review of histopathologic findings. Journal of the American Academy of Dermatology. 1990;**22**:1088-1090

[36] Ting W, Silverman NA, Arzouman DA, Levitsky S. Splenic septic emboli in endocarditis. Circulation. 1990;**82**: 105-109

[37] Scheld WM, Sande MA. Endocarditis and intravascular infections. In: Mandell GL, Bennett JE, Dolin R, editors. Mandell, Douglas and Bennett's Principles and practice of Infectious Diseases. New York: Churchill Livingstone; 1995. pp. 740-783

[38] Murdoch DR, Corey GR, Hoen B, et al. Clinical presentation, etiology, and outcome of infective endocarditis in the 21st century: The International Collaboration on Endocarditis-Prospective Cohort Study. Archives of Internal Medicine. 2009;**169**:463-473

[39] Bai AD et al. Diagnostic accuracy of transthoracic echocardiography for infective endocarditis findings using transesophageal echocardiography as the reference standard: A meta-analysis. Journal of the American Society of Echocardiography. 2017;**30**:639

[40] Michael JRMD et al. Right-sided valvular endocarditis: Etiology, diagnosis, and an approach to therapy. American Heart Journal. 1986;**111**(1): 128-135. DOI: 10.1016/0002-8703(86) 90564-8

[41] Bonow RO, Carabello BA, Chatterjee K, de Leon A, Faxon DP, Freed MD, et al. 2008 Focused update incorporated into the ACC/AHA 2006 guidelines for the management of patients with valvular heart disease: A report of the American College of Cardiology/American Heart Association Task Force on Practice Guidelines (writing committee to revise the 1998 guidelines for the management of patients with valvular heart disease). Circulation. 2008;**118**:e523-e661. DOI: 10.1161/CIRCULATIONAHA.108.190748

[42] DreyfusG SA, JebaraVA DA, ChauvaudS CJP, Carpentier A. Valve repair in acute endocarditis. The Annals of Thoracic Surgery. 1990;**49**(5): 706-711; discussion 712–3

[43] Ferringa HH, Shaw LJ, Poldermans D, Hoeks S, van der Wall EE, Dion RA, et al. Mitral valve repair and replacement in endocarditis: A systemic review of literature. The Annals of Thoracic Surgery. 2007;**83**:564-571

[44] Mervyn S, Clifford SD, Christopher WS, et al. The third international consensus definitions for sepsis and septic shock (sepsis-3). Journal of the American Medical Association. 2016;**23**: 801-810

[45] Shankar-Hari M, Phillips GS, Levy ML, Seymour CW, Liu VX, Deutschman CS, et al. Developing a new definition and assessing new clinical criteria for septic shock: For the third international consensus definitions for sepsis and septic shock (sepsis-3). Journal of the American Medical Association. 2016;**23**: 775-787

[46] Sørensen TI, Nielsen GG, Andersen PK, Teasdale TW. Genetic and environmental influences on premature death in adult adoptees. The New England Journal of Medicine. 1988;**24**: 727-732

[47] Tumangger H, Jamil K. Contribution of genes polymorphism to susceptibility and outcome of sepsis. The Egyptian Journal of Medical Human Genetics. 2010;**11**:97-103

[48] Brookes AJ. The essence of SNPs. Gene. 1999;**8**:177-186

[49] Yuzhalin AE, Kutikhin AG. Integrative systems of genomic risk markers for cancer and other diseases: Future of predictive medicine. Cancer Management and Research. 2012;**4**: 131-135

[50] Eigler A, Sinha B, Hartmann G, Endres S. Taming TNF: Strategies to restrain this proinflammatory cytokine. Immunology Today. 1997;**18**:487-492

[51] Zhang Y, Cui X, Ning L, Wei D. The effects of tumor necrosis factor-α (TNF-α) rs1800629 and rs361525 polymorphisms on sepsis risk. Oncotarget. 2017;**8**:111456-111469

[52] Delongui F, Carvalho CM, Ehara MA, Morimoto HK, Bonametti AM, Maeda JM, et al. Association of tumor necrosis factor β genetic polymorphism and sepsis susceptibility. Experimental and Therapeutic Medicine. 2011;**2**: 349-356

[53] Gómez-Jiménez J, Martín MC, Sauri R, Segura RM, Esteban F, Ruiz JC, et al. Interleukin-10 and the monocyte/macrophage-induced inflammatory response in septic shock. The Journal of Infectious Diseases. 1995; **171**:472-475

[54] Stanilova SA, Karakolev ZT, Dimov GS, Dobreva ZG, Miteva LD, Slavov ES, et al. High interleukin 12 and low interleukin 10 production after in vitro stimulation detected in sepsis survivors. Intensive Care Medicine. 2005;**31**: 401-407

[55] Stanilova SA, Miteva LD, Karakolev ZT, Stefanov CS. Interleukin-10-1082 promoter polymorphism in association with cytokine production and sepsis susceptibility. Intensive Care Medicine. 2006;**32**:260-266

[56] Dinarello CA. Immunological and inflammatory functions of the interleukin-1 family. Annual Review of Immunology. 2009;**27**:519-550

[57] Arnalich F, López-Maderuelo D, Codoceo R, Lopez J, Solis-Garrido LM, Capiscol C, et al. Interleukin-1 receptor antagonist gene polymorphism and mortality in patients with severe sepsis. Clinical and Experimental Immunology. 2002;**127**:331-336

[58] Dumitriu IE, Baruah P, Manfredi AA, Bianchi ME, Rovere-Querini P. HMGB1: Guiding immunity from within. Trends in Immunology. 2005; **26**:381-387

[59] Kornblit B, Munthe-Fog L, Madsen HO. Association of HMGB1 polymorphisms with outcome in patients with systemic inflammatory response syndrome. Critical Care. 2008; **12**:R83

[60] Jo EK. Mycobacterial interaction with innate receptors: TLRs, C-type lectins, and NLRs. Current Opinion in Infectious Diseases. 2008;**21**:279-286

[61] Mansell A, Brint E, Gould JA, O'Neill LA, Hertzog PJ. Mal interacts with tumor necrosis factor receptor-associated factor (TRAF)-6 to mediate NF-kappaB activation by toll-like receptor (TLR)-2 and TLR4. The Journal of Biological Chemistry. 2004;**279**: 37227-37230

[62] Gao JW, Zhang A, Wang X, Li Z, Yang J, Zeng L, et al. Association between the TLR2 Arg753Gln polymorphism and the risk of sepsis: A meta-analysis. Critical Care. 2015;**19**:416

[63] Rautanen A, Mills TC, Gordon AC, Hutton P, Steffens M, Nuamah R, et al. Genome-wide association study of survival from sepsis due to pneumonia: An observational cohort study. The Lancet Respiratory Medicine. 2015;**3**: 53-60

[64] Hoen B, Duval X. Epidemiology of infective endocarditis. La Revue du Praticien. 2010;**62**:511-514

[65] Golovkin AS, Ponasenko AV, Yuzhalin AE, Salakhov RR, Khutornaya MV, Kutikhin AG, et al. An association between single nucleotide polymorphisms within TLR and TREM-1 genes and infective endocarditis. Cytokine. 2015;**71**:16-21

[66] Moreau K, Clemenceau A, Le Moing V, Messika-Zeitoun D, Andersen PS, Bruun NE, et al. Human genetic susceptibility to native valve *Staphylococcus aureus* endocarditis in patients with *S. aureus* bacteremia: Genome-wide association study. Frontiers in Microbiology. 2018;**9**:640

[67] Anderson S, Bankier AT, Barrell BG, de Bruijn MH, Coulson AR, Drouin J, et al. Sequence and organization of the human mitochondrial genome. Nature. 1981;**290**:457-465

[68] Palmer J, Tandler B, Hoppel C. Biochemical properties of subsarcolemmal and interfibrillar mitochondria isolated from rat cardiac muscle. The Journal of Biological Chemistry. 1977;**252**:8731-8739

[69] Mitchell P. Coupling of phosphorylation to electron and hydrogen transfer by a chemiosmotic type of mechanism. Nature. 1961;**191**: 423-427

[70] Victor Rodwel et al. The respiratory chain & oxidative phosphorylation. Harper's Illustrated Biochemistry (103-113). New York: Mc Graw Hill; 2015

[71] Ian L, Pflugers SK. Mitochondrial function as a determinant of life span. Archiv European Journal of Physiology. 2010;**459**:277-289. DOI: 10.1007/s00424-009-0724-5

[72] Grigolava IV, Ksenzenko M, Konstantinob AA, Tikhonov AN, Kerimov TM. Tiron as a spin-trap for superoxide radicals produced by the respiratory chain of submitochondrial particles. Biokhimiia. 1980;**45**:75-82

[73] Turrens JF, Boveris A. Generation of superoxide anion by the NADH dehydrogenase of bovine heart mitochondria. The Biochemical Journal. 1980;**191**:421-427

[74] Liu Y, Fiskum G, Schubert D. Generation of reactive oxygen species by the mitochondrial electron transport chain. Journal of Neurochemistry. 2002; **80**:780-787

[75] Rich PR, Bonner WD. The sites of superoxide anion generation in higher plant mitochondria. Archives of Biochemistry and Biophysics. 1978;**188**: 206-213

[76] Klebanoff SJ. Oxygen metabolism and the toxic properties of phagocytes. Annals of Internal Medicine. 1980;**93**: 480-489

[77] Thannickal VJ, Fanburg BL. Reactive oxygen species in cell signaling. American Journal of Physiology. Lung Cellular and Molecular Physiology. 2000;**279**:L1005-L1028

[78] Han D, Antunes F, Canali R, Rettori D, Cadenas E. Voltage-dependent anion channels control the release of the superoxide anion from mitochondria to cytosol. The Journal of Biological Chemistry. 2003;**278**:5557-5563

[79] Liochev SI, Fridovich I. The Haber-Weiss cycle—70 years later: An alternative view. Redox Report. 2002; **7**(1):55-57. DOI: 10.1179/135100002125000190

[80] Zelko I, Mariani TJ, Folz RJ. Superoxide dismutase multigene family: A comparison of the CuZn-SOD (SOD1), Mn-SOD (SOD2), and EC-SOD (SOD3) gene structures, evolution, and expression. Free Radical Biology and Medicine. 2002;**33**(3):337-349. DOI: 10.1016/S0891-5849 (02)00905-X

[81] Lambeth JD. Nox enzymes, ROS, a nd chronic disease: An example of antag onistic pleiotropy. Free Radical Biology and Medicine. 2007;**43**(3):332-347

[82] Hoffman JIE, Buckberg GD. The myocardial oxygen supply: Demand index revisited. Journal of the American Heart Association. 2014;**3**:e000285

[83] Al Ghouleh I et al. Oxidases and peroxidases in cardiovascular and lung disease: New concepts in reactive oxygen species signaling. Free Radical Biology and Medicin. 2011;**51**(7): 1271-1288. DOI: 10.1016/j.freeradbiomed.2011.06.011

[84] Borchi E, Bargelli V, Stillitano F, et al. Enhanced ROS production by NADPH oxidase is correlated to changes in antioxidant enzyme activity in human heart failure. Biochimica et Biophysica Acta. 2010;**1802**:331-338

[85] Kuroda J, Ago T, Matsushima S, Zhai P, Schneider MD, Sadoshima J. NADPH oxidase 4 (Nox4) is a major source of oxidative stress in the failing heart. Proceedings of the National Academy of Sciences of the United States of America. 2010;**107**: 15565-15570

[86] Ide T, Tsutsui H, Kinugawa S, et al. Direct evidence for increased hydroxyl radicals originating from superoxide in the failing myocardium. Circulation Research. 2000;**86**:152-157

[87] Moreillon P, Que YA. Infective endocarditis. Lancet. 2004;**363**:139-149

[88] Ostrowski S et al. Myocardial oxidative stress in patients with active infective endocarditis. International Journal of Cardiology. 15 Jul 2013;**167** (1):270-276. DOI: 10.1016/j.ijcard.2011.12.102. PubMed PMID: 22244479. [Epub 2012 Jan 13]

[89] Wu F, Tyml K, Wilson JX. iNOS expression requires NADPH oxidase-dependent redox signaling in microvascular endothelial cells. Journal of Cellular Physiology. 2008;**217**(1): 207-214. DOI: 10.1002/jcp.21495

[90] Langley RJ, Tsalik EL, van Velkinburgh JC, et al. An integrated clinico-metabolomic model improves prediction of death in sepsis. Science Translational Medicine. 2013;**5**(195): 195ra95. DOI: 10.1126/scitranslmed.3005893

[91] Lee CF et al. Normalization of NAD + redox balance as a therapy for heart failure. Circulation. 2016;**134**: 883-894. DOI: 10.1161/CIRCULATIONAHA.116.022495

[92] Jones S, Holm T, Mager I, Langel U, Howl J. Characterization of bioactive cell penetrating peptides from human cytochrome c: Protein mimicry and the development of a novel apoptogenic agent. Chemistry & Biology. 2010;**17**: 735-744

[93] Piel DA, Deutschman CS, Levy RJ. Exogenous cytochrome C restores myocardial cytochrome oxidase activity into the late phase of sepsis. Shock. 2008;**29**:612-616

[94] Piel DA, Gruber PJ, Weinheimer CJ, Courtois MR, Robertson CM, Coopersmith CM, et al. Mitochondrial resuscitation with exogenous

cytochrome c in the septic heart. Critical Care Medicine. 2007;**35**:2120-2127

[95] Hotchkiss RS et al. Apoptotic cell death in patients with sepsis, shock, and multiple organ dysfunction. Critical Care Medicine. 1999 Jul;**27**(7):1230-1251

[96] Chung CS, Chaudry IH, Ayala A. The apoptotic response of the lymphoid immune system to trauma, shock and sepsis. In: Vincent J-L, editor. Yearbook of Intensive Care and Emergency Medicine. Berlin: Spinger-Verlag; 2000. pp. 27-40

[97] Hotchkiss RS, Swanson PE, Freeman BD, Tinsley KW, Cobb JP, Matuschak GM, et al. Apoptotic cell death in patients with sepsis, shock and multiple organ dysfunction. Critical Care Medicine. 1999;**27**:1230-1251

[98] Hotchkiss RS, et al. Accelerated lymphocyte death in sepsis occurs by both the death receptor and mitochondrial pathways. Journal of Immunology. 2005;**174**(8):5110-5118

[99] Hiramatsu M, Hotchkiss RS, Karl IE, Buchman TG. Cecal ligation and puncture (CLP) induces apoptosis in thymus, spleen, lung, and gut by an endotoxin and TNF-independent pathway. Shock. 1997;7:247-253

[100] Mesotten D, Swinnen JV, Vanderhoydonc F, Wouters P, van den Berghe G. Contribution of circulating lipids to the improved outcome of critical illness by glycemic control with intensive insulin therapy. Journal of Clinical Endocrinology & Metabolism. 2004;**89**:219-226

[101] Andersen SK, Gjedsted J, Christiansen C, Tonnesen E. The roles of insulin and hyperglycemia in sepsis pathogenesis. Journal of Leukocyte Biology. 2004;**75**:413-421

[102] Giraldo FA. Epidemiology of Infective Endocarditis. En Contemporary Challenges in Endocar ditis (35-55). DOI: 10.5772/ 65030

[103] Clark MF, Baudouin SV. A systematic review of the quality of genetic association studies in human sepsis. Intensive Care Medicine. 2006; **32**(11):1706-1712

[104] Foteinou PT et al, Model for the assessment of autonomic dysfunction in human endotoxemia. Physiol Genomics. 2010;**42**(1):5-19. PMID: 20233835

[105] Foteinou PT, Calvano SE, Lowry SF, Androulakis IP. Translational potential of systems-based models of inflammation [thesis]. Clinical and Translational Science. 2008;**2**(1):85-89

[106] Pedro E. Alvarado Rubio et al. Loss of Complexity of the Cardiac Bioelectrical Signal as an Expression of Patient Outcomes. Interpreting Cardiac Electrograms (169-182). DOI: 10.5772/ intechopen.70144

Chapter 6

Non-bacterial Thrombotic Endocarditis

Carmen Busca-Arenzana, Angel Robles-Marhuenda, Luis Ramos-Ruperto and Jorge Alvarez-Troncoso

Abstract

Non-bacterial thrombotic endocarditis or also called verrucous endocarditis or Libman-Sacks endocarditis or marantic endocarditis is a rare entity, still unknown physiopathology, which is characterized by the formation of sterile vegetations at the valvular structures. These vegetations of platelet aggregates and fibrin are sterile by definition, so for its definitive diagnosis, it is essential to rule out an infectious endocarditis. It is mainly diagnosed by echocardiography in patients with neoplasms or systemic autoimmune diseases. Its main complication is the formation of multi-systemic embolisms, preferably at the brain level, so anticoagulation will be fundamental in the treatment and evolution of non-bacterial thrombotic endocarditis.

Keywords: Libman-Sacks endocarditis, marantic endocarditis, non-bacterial thrombotic endocarditis, non-infective endocarditis, verrucous endocarditis

1. Introduction

Non-bacterial thrombotic endocarditis (NBTE) is a rare entity in which a state of hypercoagulability predisposes to the formation of sterile vegetations in heart valves and secondary systemic embolisms, mainly in the central nervous system. In many occasions, the diagnosis is made postmortem, finding up to 0.2% of the autopsies of the general population [1]. The pathogenesis is unknown, being associated mainly with the existence of neoplastic processes and systemic autoimmune diseases (mainly in systemic lupus erythematosus (SLE) or antiphospholipid syndrome (APS)).

For the diagnosis it is necessary to demonstrate the presence of valvular vegetations by echocardiography, ruling out the existence of an underlying infection. There is no specific treatment, so it is recommended to control the predisposing disease and the initiation of anticoagulation to avoid the production of systemic embolisms [2].

2. Epidemiology and etiology

The NBTE is a rare pathology, whose diagnosis occurs generally in autopsies, being present in 0.9–1.2% of them, according to the series [3]. However, it is believed to be an underdiagnosed entity. It is described at any age, although it is more prevalent in patients between 40 and 80 years of age. Children tend to present milder clinical forms, with a lower number of systemic embolisms [4].

a. Malignancy • Mucin-secreting and pancreatic adenocarcinoma • Lung malignant neoplasm • Ovary carcinoma • Colon carcinoma • Prostate carcinoma • Cholangiocarcinoma • Lymphoma
b. Systemic autoimmune diseases • Systemic lupus erythematosus • Antiphospholipid syndrome • Systemic vasculitis ° Giant cell arteritis ° Behçet disease ° Takayasu's arteritis ° Polyangiitis with granulomatosis
c. Hypercoagulability states • Protein S and C deficiency • Disseminated intravascular coagulation • Thrombotic microangiopathy ° Thrombotic thrombocytopenic purpura ° Catastrophic antiphospholipid syndrome
d. Chronic inflammatory status • Tuberculosis • Uncontrolled HIV • Chronic pyelonephritis • Chronic osteomyelitis
e. Others • Adenomyosis • Hypereosinophilic syndrome • Chronic alcoholism • Chronic renal insufficiency • Heart failure with valvulopathy • Toxic oil syndrome

Table 1.
Causes of NBTE.

The neoplastic disease, generally advanced, is the main risk factor for the development of NBTE. If compared with the general population, this subgroup has a higher risk of presenting it (1.25 vs. 0.2%, respectively) according to a series of autopsies [5, 6]. The adenocarcinomas (i.e., colon, ovary, lung) are the most frequent tumors, observing a greater number of cases in the pancreatic and mucin secretors. Other pathologies that are associated are the SLE and the APS. In the SLE, different observational studies show a prevalence ranging between 6 and 11%, being more frequent among lupus patients with antiphospholipid antibodies [7]. Although exceptionally, NBTE can be a complication of systemic infections such as tuberculosis and HIV, and cases have been described in the context of uremia, adenomyosis, and even giant cell arteritis [8]. It should be said that in the cases mentioned of infectious etiology (i.e., tuberculosis, HIV), the development of NBTE is not determined directly by microorganisms, but by alterations in coagulation induced by the underlying chronic inflammatory process (**Table 1**).

3. Pathogenesis

NBTE is a type of noninfectious endocarditis whose physiopathology continues to be unknown. It is characterized by the deposition of sterile platelet thrombi in the heart valves. In certain situations of hypercoagulability, endothelial damage occurs that favors the migration of mononuclear inflammatory cells and platelet deposition, being these responsible for the formation of fibrin thrombi and immune complexes (thrombi known as "white thrombus"). The term Libman-Sacks is used when you see a large thrombus or "wart" (verrucous endocarditis).

One of the main and differential characteristics of this entity is that the valvular vegetations must always be sterile (unlike infectious endocarditis (IE)). The mitral and aortic valves are the most frequently affected (rare right endocarditis), and it is common for NBTE to appear on healthy native valves, endocardium, or chordae tendineae.

Unlike IE, vegetations of the NBTE are more friable because they develop on a tissue with an important inflammatory reaction. This makes them more likely to produce systemic embolisms. They are located in the valvular coaptation lines and

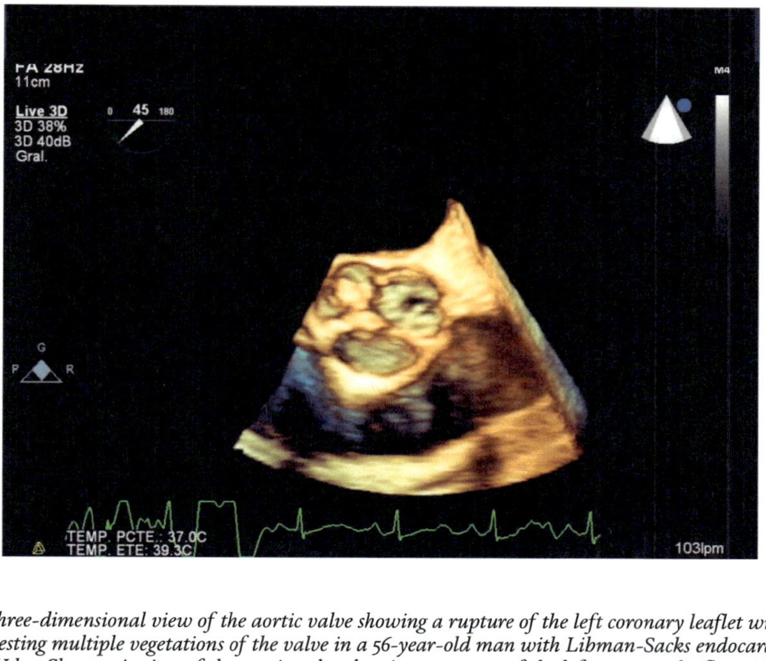

Figure 1.
ETE-3D: Three-dimensional view of the aortic valve showing a rupture of the left coronary leaflet with images suggesting multiple vegetations of the valve in a 56-year-old man with Libman-Sacks endocarditis and SLE. ETE-Velos: Short axis view of the aortic valve showing a rupture of the left coronary leaflet with images suggesting thickening and multiple vegetations in the leaflets.

are generally not accompanied by destruction of the valvular tissue. In terms of their size, they tend to be smaller and develop on a broad and irregular basis [9].

In NBTEs associated with malignancy, it is believed that macrophages interact with tumor cells, causing a migration of cytokines (tumor necrosis factor, interleukin-1, etc.) that produces endothelial tissue damage and the formation of friable thrombi due to the deposition of platelets. On the other hand, the macrophage-tumor cell interaction favors overactivation of the coagulation cascade, which in turn worsens the state of hypercoagulability that underlies the process. For this reason, NBTE tends to develop around areas of greater valve turbulence [3].

Libman-Sacks endocarditis is the most characteristic cardiac manifestation of SLE, with pericarditis being the most frequent cardiac manifestation [10]. It was first described in 1924, by Libman and Sacks at Mount Sinai Hospital in New York. From the macroscopic point of view, these deposits, usually located on the ventricular surface of the posterior leaflet of the mitral valve, are translated into vegetations with progressive growth or only thickening of the leaflets (**Figure 1**). The classic histopathological lesion consists of a deposit of fibrin and mononuclear cells. The immunofluorescence reveals immunoglobulin deposit and complement. Valvular involvement is usually silent and occurs in approximately half of patients with SLE, although in some cases valvular dysfunction can be the origin of heart failure. As in other NBTEs, the mitral and aortic valves are affected more frequently than those on the right side, with valvular insufficiency prevailing over the stenosis. The presence of lupus anticoagulant increases the risk of suffering thrombotic and embolic phenomena in these patients [11].

4. Clinical presentation

NBTE is characterized as an asymptomatic disease in early stages, whose most frequent initial manifestation is the presence of systemic embolisms. Although it can occur at any age, it is believed that young patients are less likely to suffer from embolic phenomena at a distance.

The clinic of valvular dysfunction (in the form of heart failure, syncope, etc.) usually appears in more advanced stages of the disease, and although it is recognizable by echocardiographic studies, they usually have little hemodynamic repercussion, except in advanced cases or the presence of large masses. The development of heart failure is present in less than half of patients with underlying valvular dysfunction.

4.1 Characteristics of embolisms

Given the rarity of this entity, the incidence of embolisms at the systemic level is not known. It is believed that it can appear from 14 to 91% of the NBTE. The embolisms, some with hemorrhagic transformation, are more frequent in cases associated with malignancy [12]. In these patients, embolisms are evident in up to 50% of the cases, the most frequent clinical form being the central nervous system involvement.

Patients with NBTE usually debut in the form of multiple embolisms, especially distributed throughout the brain territory in the form of multiple infarcts (sometimes casual diagnosis after performing brain imaging tests). This contrasts with IE, where typically infarcts are usually focal and/or localized.

4.2 Signs and symptoms

Most patients are asymptomatic during the early stages of the disease. In fact, the appearance of fever, weight loss, and night sweats is uncommon, and its presence should guide us in the search for an underlying neoplastic process. On the other hand,

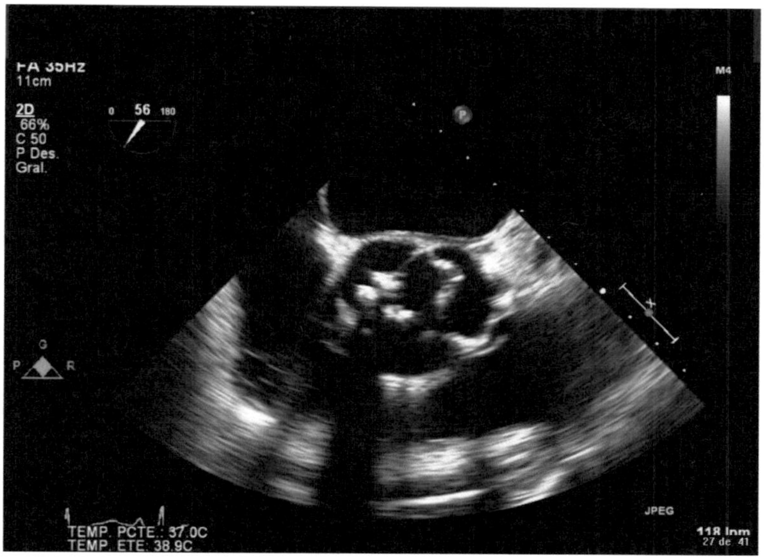

Figure 2.
ETT-IM: Four-chamber color view showing a jet of severe mitral regurgitation in a 48-year-old man with catastrophic antiphospholipid syndrome.

the association of arthritis, photosensitive skin lesions, and arterial and/or venous thromboses requires screening for systemic autoimmune diseases (SLE or APS).

The typical form of presentation (in more than half of the cases) derives from the symptoms and signs that occur as a result of the presence of systemic embolisms. Although they can be produced in different organs (CNS, kidney, spleen, skin, etc.), in 50% of cases, embolisms are observed at the pulmonary level, sometimes in the absence of valvular lesions in right cardiac cavities [13].

Sometimes the symptoms may be mild or nonspecific, such as hematuria, lumbar pain, and rash, in the context of renal, splenic, or cutaneous embolisms, respectively. However, the presence of coronary and CNS lesions is more specific and helps the diagnosis more early (chest pain, psychomotor agitation, delirium, stroke, etc.). The debut in the form of valvular insufficiency or decompensated heart failure is very infrequent [14] (**Figure 2**).

5. Diagnosis

The diagnosis of NBTE is a challenge for the clinician (which is why it is often diagnosed after carrying out necropsies) and not only due to the lack of specificity of the clinic but also because it occurs in advanced stages of the disease.

The diagnosis of NBTE is made through a high clinical suspicion after observing systemic manifestations derived from systemic embolisms and after performing complementary imaging tests (echocardiogram and transesophageal echocardiography mainly) that confirm the presence of valvular vegetations. However, the definitive diagnosis can be obtained after histologically demonstrating the presence of platelet thrombi at the level of the cardiac valves. It is a rare phenomenon, since valvular biopsies are not performed routinely. For this, it is essential to rule out the presence of a systemic infection and to identify the underlying etiology (mainly autoimmune neoplasms and diseases).

It is necessary to make a correct differential diagnosis that includes IE, degenerative valvular disease, rheumatic valvular disease, and normal anatomic variants. Applying the modified Duke's criteria can help establish the IE diagnosis [15].

Therefore, we should suspect an NBTE in those patients with active neoplasia, SLE or, APS who present coronary or CNS ischemia or, in the absence of said predisposing pathologies, in those cases in which we suspect an IE (without microbiological findings) that does not respond adequately directed empirical antibiotic treatment and that evolves torpidly with a greater number of systemic embolisms.

5.1 Laboratory and microbiology test

There are no specific analytical tests that suggest the presence of an NBTE. Depending on the causative disease, we can find analytical alterations that support or not a diagnosis. A complete blood test should be performed, including blood count, biochemistry, liver test, and coagulation panel. In some patients with NBTE, data of disseminated intravascular coagulation can be evidenced. In case of suspicion of autoimmune disease, a complete immunological study should be requested, mainly from SLE and APS (including antinuclear antibody, anti-double-stranded DNA, and antiphospholipid antibodies). It will be necessary to carry out a screening of the most frequent types of neoplasms taking into account the sex, the comorbidities, and the age range of the patient.

Many authors suggest that before diagnosing an NBTE, it is essential to rule out an IE after carrying out different microbiological tests. In fact, at least three sets of blood cultures must be made before any suspicion of IE. Sometimes blood cultures in the presence of valvular vegetations can be persistently negative and do not rule out the presence of IE (called "culture-negative endocarditis"). For this reason, cultures of other biological fluids (urine, feces, etc.) should be performed, and serology and PCR should be performed on those less frequent or "atypical" microorganisms that can also cause IE (e.g., *Brucella* spp., *Coxiella burnetii*, *Legionella*, etc.) (**Table 2**).

5.2 Radiological image tests

The performance of radiological image tests will depend on the symptomatology that the patient presents, since they will provide information in those cases of complicated NBTE. In chest X-ray, we can observe data that suggest heart failure (cardiomegaly, pleural effusion, etc.). Cranial computed tomography (CT) and magnetic resonance (MR) imaging are very useful for the diagnosis of cerebral embolisms, since if we suspect an NBTE, multiple infarcts will be observed, widely distributed, heterogeneous in size, and mainly ischemic. Cardiac MR or positron emission tomography may help in the differential diagnosis.

1. Previous antibiotic treatment
2. Technical problems with microbiological diagnosis
3. Acute renal failure or renal insufficiency
4. Ventricular or atrial septal defects, cardiac thrombi post-acute coronary disease, or cardiac pacemaker infection
5. Unusual microorganisms (*Brucella* spp., *Coxiella burnetii*, *Bartonella* spp., *Legionella* spp., *Mycoplasma* spp., *Tropheryma whipplei*, mycotic infections, and HACEK group infections—*Haemophilus* spp., *Aggregatibacter* spp., *Cardiobacterium hominis*, *Eikenella corrodens*, and *Kingella* species)

Table 2.
Culture-negative endocarditis causes.

5.3 Echocardiography

In those patients with suspected NBTE, a two-dimensional transthoracic echocardiography (TTE) should be performed to demonstrate the presence of vegetations or valvular thickening (**Figure 3**). Vegetations in the NBTE usually appear in left valves, with the mitral valve most frequently affected (up to 75% of cases) followed by the aortic valve. Several valves can be affected simultaneously, although it is usually an uncommon finding (**Figure 4**).

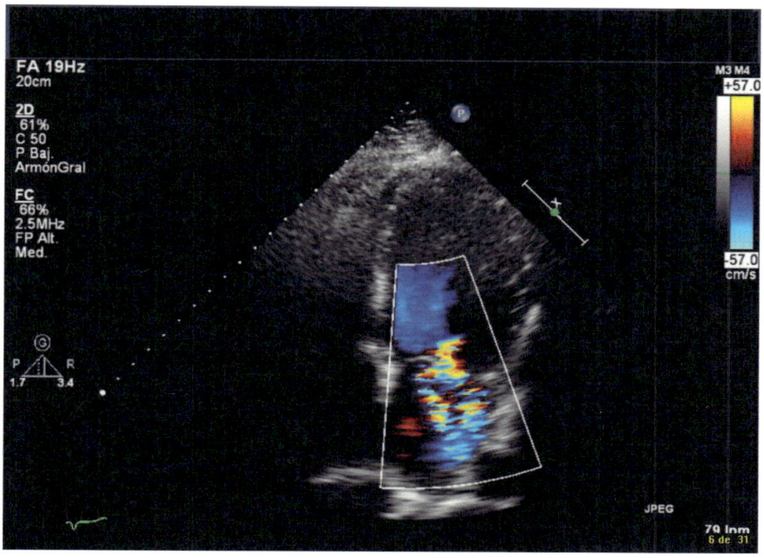

Figure 3.
ETE-2C: Mid-esophageal two-chamber view showing a 28-mm vegetation in the mitral valve.

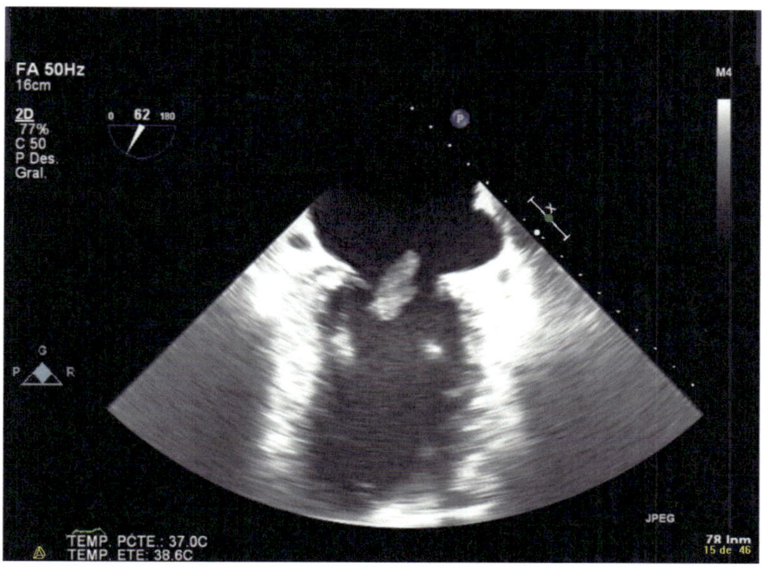

Figure 4.
ETE-2C: Mid-esophageal two-chamber color view. A vegetation in the mitral valve can be visualized. A severe mitral regurgitation jet is shown in this figure.

However, TTE has several limitations. Small vegetations (below 5 mm) may go unnoticed, so if the clinical suspicion is still high, there is an indication to perform a transesophageal echocardiography (TEE), since it is more sensitive and specific than the TTE in detecting smaller vegetations. Do not forget that very small vegetations (<3 mm) cannot be detected by both types of echocardiogram, being able to obtain "false negatives." If the clinical suspicion persists, echocardiographic study should be repeated after a prudential time. Although TTE is less sensitive and specific than TEE, it should always be performed not only to confirm the presence of endocarditis but also to evaluate other fundamental parameters such as function and cardiac volumes.

Although the echocardiogram is essential in the diagnosis of valvular vegetations, it will not be useful for the differential diagnosis of the type of endocarditis (thrombotic infection vs. aggregations of platelets and fibrin).

5.4 Histology

Although the definitive diagnosis is histological, most of the anatomopathological tests of valvular vegetations are obtained from necropsies or after valve replacement after the finding of a severe dysfunction or insufficiency, being very rare the biopsies of tendinous, valvular cords, or endocardial.

6. Treatment and management

There is no specific treatment for NBTE. The two basic pillars are systemic anticoagulation and targeted specific treatment of the associated disease (chemotherapy, corticosteroids, etc.). In general, surgery by means of intervention, debridement, or valve replacement is usually not necessary and is rarely indicated.

6.1 Anticoagulation

Anticoagulant treatment is essential in the management of NBTE since it aims to prevent the production of systemic embolisms. In fact, unlike EI, these patients have an indication for anticoagulation for long periods of time or even indefinitely (unless absolutely contraindicated), regardless of whether embolic phenomena are observed or not. This fact is based on the fragility of the vegetations and the recurrent tendency to systemic embolization, especially in the absence of antithrombotic therapy. It should always be anticoagulated with a double objective: preventive and therapeutic. There are no published randomized clinical trials or prospective studies, so the recommendations are based on case series and retrospective studies and are supported by the American College of Chest Physician's antithrombotic therapy for valvular heart disease guidelines [16].

Anticoagulation will be carried out by subcutaneous low molecular weight heparin or intravenous unfractionated heparin at anticoagulant doses. All the evidence published to date supports the use of this pharmacological family and does not recommend the use of warfarin, direct thrombin, nor factor Xa inhibitor (direct oral anticoagulants like apixaban, rivaroxaban, dabigatran, or edoxaban) especially in patients with active neoplastic disease since they seem to have less efficacy in the reduction of systemic embolisms. There is no data to support the use of the new anticoagulants. Recently the first case of cancer-associated non-bacterial thrombotic endocarditis in the era of direct oral anticoagulants was published where a patient with a previous history of thromboembolic disease developed a NBTE with vegetations and multiple cerebral embolisms in the context of a pancreatic adenocarcinoma despite being under treatment with rivaroxaban at optimal doses [17]. This case supports the need to carry out more studies that help to elucidate the physiopathogenic mechanisms of the NBTE with the aim of achieving an optimal anticoagulant regimen.

The most frequent complications are life-threatening bleeding and thrombocytopenia. The development of any of these complications will force clinicians to raise the risk-benefit of their use and therefore to value discontinuing their use.

6.2 Surgery

In general, indications for valve replacement or vegetation excision are very limited in the NBTE. The main objective of surgery in the NBTE is to reduce or prevent the production of systemic embolisms. Because there are no prospective clinical trials, the same recommendations should be followed as in patients with IE [18].

However, unlike IE, we will try to preserve the valve as much as possible and focus all the objectives in controlling the state of hypercoagulability by treating predisposing disease.

When deciding whether a patient is going to benefit from surgery, it is essential to assess the risk-benefit individually. The surgical repair of heart valve is preferable (it is less aggressive, has less mortality, and in general decreases the need for postoperative anticoagulation), with respect to valve replacement. The latter will be considered depending on the complications and the degree of destruction or valvular insufficiency. We must take into account the prognosis of life and morbidity and mortality, especially in patients with advanced neoplastic diseases. Although there is little evidence, it is believed that anticoagulation should be maintained after surgery, especially in patients with systemic autoimmune diseases (mainly in APS).

6.3 Treatment for underlying disease

The treatment of neoplasia or systemic autoimmune disease is a fundamental pillar in the management of NBTE. It is very probable that at the time of diagnosis of the neoplasm, distant metastases are already observed, which will considerably reduce the probability of therapeutic success. The same is not true in patients with SLE, where NBTE can be diagnosed at any time and whose presence does not correlate with the activity index. The treatment of patients with lupus valve disease includes prophylaxis of endocarditis, antiplatelet or anticoagulant treatment in selected cases, and valvular replacement when valvular involvement is severe; the role of corticosteroid treatment in the evolution of valvular disease is still undetermined. Regarding the type of surgical intervention, there are controversies. Some authors suggest the superiority of mechanical prostheses in this type of condition over bioprostheses, including cryopreserved homografts, as these can contract lupus valvulitis on the new valve. However, other authors have advocated reconstructive surgery to avoid the disadvantages of a mechanical prosthesis in young patients who usually require high doses of steroids and anticoagulant therapy [19].

It is unknown whether NBTE improves with antineoplastic therapy, and therefore it is believed that anticoagulation should be maintained independently of the response to treatment of the underlying disease.

7. Evolution and prognosis

7.1 Follow-up

The follow-up should be individualized depending on the characteristics and morbidities of each patient. It will be necessary to take into account possible complications of the disease or treatment: systemic embolization, bleeding, or thrombocytopenia. It will be necessary to periodically perform echocardiograms to monitor valve function, control the development of new vegetations (or check their resolution), as well as monitor the appearance of an IE concomitantly.

7.2 Prognosis

The prognosis of NBTE has not been correctly evaluated in prospective studies. In general, the prognosis of these patients is poor, although it will depend on the type of disease and the type or location of the complications, independently of the anticoagulant treatment.

8. Conclusions

- The NBTE is an entity characterized by the presence of vegetations of noninfectious origin constituted by fibrin and platelet accumulations with high emboligenic potential.
- The most frequent etiologies are neoplasms (especially carcinoma of the pancreas) in an advanced or disseminated phase, without forgetting the systemic immune-mediated processes such as lupus.
- Embolism and valvular dysfunction are the two most frequent complications found in NBTE. The incidence of systemic embolisms is around 50% in malignant NTBE, with neurological manifestations being the most common.
- The therapeutic attitude in these patients should be directed toward the control of the underlying disease and the hypercoagulable state or the treatment of the embolisms.

Conflict of interest

The authors do not present any conflict of interest.

Author details

Carmen Busca-Arenzana, Angel Robles-Marhuenda*, Luis Ramos-Ruperto and Jorge Alvarez-Troncoso
Internal Medicine Department, La Paz University Hospital, Madrid, Spain

*Address all correspondence to: aroblesmarhuenda@gmail.com

References

[1] Smeglin A, Ansari M, Skali H, et al. Marantic endocarditis and disseminated intravascular coagulation with systemic emboli in presentation of pancreatic cancer. Journal of Clinical Oncology. 2008;**26**:1383-1385

[2] Liu J, Frishman WH. Nonbacterial thrombotic endocarditis, pathogenesis, diagnosis and management. Cardiology in Review. 2016;**24**:5

[3] Bauer KA. Nonbacterial thrombotic endocarditis. Uptodate; 2018

[4] Sharma J, Lasic Z, Bornstein A, et al. Libman-Sacks endocarditis as the first manifestation of systemic lupus erythematosus in an adolescent, with a review of the literature. Cardiology in the Young. 2013;**23**:1-6

[5] Rosen P, Armstrong D. Nonbacterial thrombotic endocarditis in patients with malignant neoplastic diseases. The American Journal of Medicine. 1973;**54**:23

[6] González Quintela A, Candela MJ, Vidal C, et al. Non-bacterial thrombotic endocarditis in cancer patients. Acta Cardiologica. 1991;**46**:1

[7] Roldan CA, Qualls CR, Sopko KS, Sibbitt WL Jr. Transthoracic versus transesophageal echocardiography for detection of Libman-Sacks endocarditis: A randomized controlled study. The Journal of Rheumatology. 2008;**35**:224

[8] Terré A, Lidove O, Georges O, Mesnildrey P, Chennebault H, Ziza JM. Non-infective endocarditis: Expanding the phenotype of giant cell arteritis. Joint Bone Spine. 2017; article in press

[9] Roldan CA, Sibbitt WL Jr, Qualls CR, et al. Libman-Sacks endocarditis and embolic cerebrovascular disease. JACC: Cardiovascular Imaging. 2013;**6**:973

[10] Asherson RA, Gibson DG, Evans DW, Baguley E, Hughes GR. Diagnostic and therapeutic problems in two patients with antiphospholipid antibodies, heart valve lesions, and transient ischemic attacks. Annals of the Rheumatic Diseases. 1988;**47**:947-953

[11] Lee JL, Naguwa SM, Cheema GS, Gershwin ME. Revisiting Libman-Sacks endocarditis: A historical review and update. Clinical Reviews in Allergy and Immunology. 2009;**36**:126-130

[12] Edoute Y, Haim N, Rinkevich D, Brenner B, Reisner SA. Cardiac valvular vegetations in cancer patients: A prospective echocardiographic study of 200 patients. The American Journal of Medicine. 1997;**102**:252-258

[13] El-Shami K, Griffiths E, Streiff M. Nonbacterial thrombotic endocarditis in cancer patients: Pathogenesis, diagnosis, and treatment. The Oncologist. 2007;**12**:518

[14] Mazokopakis EE, Syros PK, Starakis IK. Nonbacterial thrombotic endocarditis (marantic endocarditis) in cancer patients. Cardiovascular and Hematological Disorders Drug Targets. 2010;**10**:84

[15] Li JS, Sexton DJ, Mick N, et al. Proposed modifications to the Duke criteria for the diagnosis of infective endocarditis. Clinical Infectious Diseases. 2000;**30**:633-638

[16] Whitlock RP, Sun JC, Fremes SE, et al. Antithrombotic and thrombolytic therapy for valvular disease: Antithrombotic Therapy and Prevention of Thrombosis, 9th ed: American College of Chest Physicians Evidence-Based Clinical Practice Guidelines. Chest. 2012;**141**:e576S

[17] Mantovani F, Barbieri A, Boriani G. A first described case of

cancer- associated non-bacterial thrombotic endocarditis in the era of direct oral anticoagulants. Thrombosis Research. 2017;**149**:45-47

[18] Nishimura RA, Otto CM, Bonow RO, et al. AHA/ACC guideline for the management of patients with valvular heart disease: Executive summary: A report of the American College of Cardiology/American Heart Association Task Force on Practice Guidelines. Circulation. 2014;**129**:2440-2492

[19] Fernández-Dueñas J, López-Granados A, Mesa-Rubio D, Ariza-Cañete J, Gallo-Marín M, Concha-Ruiz M. Regurgitación mitral severa en endocarditis de Libman-Sacks. Cirugía reparadora. Revista Española de Cardiología. 2005;**58**(9):1118-1120. DOI: 10.1157/13078558

Chapter 7

Cardiac Implantable Electronic Device-Related Infections

Måns Almqvist, Gustav Mattsson, Robin Razmi and Peter Magnusson

Abstract

The use of cardiac devices, that is, pacemakers and implantable cardioverter defibrillators, has increased, and the incidence will likely continue to increase due to an aging population with associated risk factors. Unfortunately, this implies an increasing number of complications, including infections. Cardiac device-related infection is a dreaded complication causing both increased morbidity and mortality, and considerable costs. Because of the presence of a foreign body in subcutaneous tissue, vasculature, and the heart, patients with cardiac device systems are at increased risk of endocarditis due to microbial agents. In general, an infected device system should be removed in its entirety. The timing of reimplantation varies due to indication and severity of the infection. Furthermore, the explant procedure may be complicated and should be performed by an experienced team including facilities to handle life-threatening complications. The subcutaneous implantable cardioverter defibrillator or leadless pacemaker can serve as an option in selected cases. This chapter will describe clinical aspects of cardiac device-related infections.

Keywords: cardiac device, endocarditis, infection, implantable cardioverter defibrillator, pacemaker

1. Introduction

Infective endocarditis (IE) is a potentially lethal disease. First described by Osler more than a century ago, it remains associated with a considerable burden of complications and death [1–3]. In fact, the incidence has increased over the years—in part reflecting a growing number of comorbidities in an aging population. Improvements in cardiovascular health care have not only contributed to increased life expectancy but also to a growing number of patients living with underlying cardiovascular pathologies that constitute risk factors for IE. Thus, endocarditis can be described as an adverse consequence of medical advances. This is certainly valid in the case of endocarditis affecting cardiac implantable electronic devices (CIEDs). Since the introduction of the pacemaker as a routine treatment for bradyarrhythmias in the 1960s, a rapid evolution of technology has resulted in several new implantable devices. CIEDs also include implantable cardioverter defibrillators (ICD) and cardiac resynchronization therapy (CRT). Today, device therapy is an essential therapeutic modality of cardiovascular care. It has extended the life span of patients and also improved health-related quality of life. Nowadays, approximately 1.2 million CIEDs are implanted each year worldwide [4].

This highly conventional and routine device treatment is however clouded by its potentially devastating complications. CIED infection is a severe complication associated with high mortality [5, 6]. The implantation rate is increasing globally and US data indicate that this is coupled with increased implantation in older patients with more co-morbidities. An increased use of more complex device systems also implies higher risks. All of this contributes to an end result of more CIED infections. As the disease panorama and indications are similar in large parts of the world, a similar increase outside the US seems inevitable.

A CIED infection can be challenging to diagnose and treat. It may involve the generator pocket, the leads, the endocardial structures, or a combination thereof. Involvement of endocardial structures including valves implies higher mortality. Diagnostic difficulties can be even greater than in IE because echocardiography is less accurate, blood cultures are less sensitive, and the diagnosis is sometimes not considered because of unspecific symptoms. Attempts to salvage infected devices are often unsuccessful. In this chapter, we present an outline of current recommendations regarding prevention, diagnostics, and management of CIED infections.

2. Technology and terminology

Cardiac device management involves many technical details. For those less familiar with these procedures, we recommend the supplementary appendix of a recent review [7]. In addition to an outline of the generators, leads, and materials used in CIEDs, it also describes the normal step-by-step procedures of implanting, revising, and removing CIEDs. Abbreviations are both abundant and inevitable in this field and are summarized at the end of this chapter.

3. Definition and categorization of CIED infection

There are no universally agreed definitions of CIED infection. Previously used definitions have varied, but common starting points have been the site or sites of infection on one hand and the signs of probable infection on the other [8, 9]. One common and theoretically simple distinction is between local device infection and infection also affecting the blood stream, leads, and/or cardiac valves. However, in clinical practice, it is sometimes difficult to differentiate between these categories [5]. The lack of a golden standard calls for a clear presentation of used criteria. Our proposed classification, summarized below, is a synthesis of earlier studies, recommendations, and guidelines [7, 10, 11].

In short, we suggest six different categories relevant when CIED infection is considered. These are presented in **Table 1**, besides basic strategies for device and antibiotic management. The first of three categories involving the generator pocket is not a definite infection but rather early post-implantation inflammation. These superficial signs of wound inflammation are expected to wear off shortly, when suspected causes such as sutures or dressing are removed. However, as they also can be an early sign of infection, close observation is recommended.

Actual infections can be categorized as complicated or uncomplicated pocket infection based on whether they also involve blood stream infection. Echocardiography and the modified Duke criteria can be used to classify more extensive infections: suspected or definite lead infection (CIED-LI), and CIED-associated infective endocarditis affecting the heart valves (CIED-IE) [12]. A large proportion of patients end up as "possible CIED-LI". Diagnosing a definite and isolated CIED-LI

Diagnostic classifications	Device an antibiotic strategy	Treatment duration***
Early post-implantation inflammation Erythema near the incision site within 30 days of implantation WITHOUT any of the following: - purulent exudate, - dehiscence, - fluctuance, - systemic signs of infection* A small area (<1 cm) of erythema and purulence next to a stich, (*stich abscess*), is also included in this category.	- No need for device extraction. - Remove suspected cause (stitches or local dressing/skin preparation) - Consider observation only or short oral empiric antibiotic therapy and expect clinical resolution within 2 weeks. Close observation as this can be early signs of pocket infection.	Consider 7–10 days of flucloxacillin. For penicillin-allergic or MRSA-colonized patients, consider clindamycin.
Pocket infection—uncomplicated One or more of the following: - spreading cellulitis around the pocket, or - incision site purulent exudate (excluding stitch abscess), or - wound dehiscence, or - erosion through skin with exposure of generator or leads,** or - fluctuance (abscess) or fistula formation AND: negative blood cultures AND: no signs of systemic infection	- Device removal recommended - Commence intravenous empiric antibiotic therapy targeting Gram-positive (including MRSA) bacteria. (Treatment for Gram-negative bacteria will depend on susceptibility testing after blood cultures for this group). - Start targeted treatment after results from blood cultures.	10–14 days iv (if no complications occur)
Pocket infection—complicated As uncomplicated pocket infection, but WITH: - positive blood cultures, or - evidence of lead or endocardial infection, or - symptoms/signs of systemic infection.	- Device removal recommended - Commence intravenous empiric antibiotic therapy targeting both Gram-positive (including MRSA) and Gram-negative bacteria. - Start targeted treatment after results from blood cultures.	Treat as CIED-IE or CIED-LI depending on the nature of complication.
Definite CIED lead infection (CIED-LI) Symptoms/signs of systemic infection NO signs of generator pocket infection AND: echocardiography consistent with lead vegetations AND: presence of major Duke microbiological criteria [12] OR: Symptoms/signs of systemic infection NO signs of generator pocket infection AND culture, histology, or molecular evidence of infection on explanted lead	- Device removal recommended - Commence intravenous empiric antibiotic therapy targeting both Gram-positive (including MRSA) and Gram-negative bacteria. - Start targeted treatment after results from blood cultures.	For isolated CIED-LI consider short course, 2 weeks of treatment after device removal. If any uncertainty (as when tricuspid valve is not normal or "ghost lesions" remain after device removal): treat as CIED-IE.

Diagnostic classifications	Device an antibiotic strategy	Treatment duration***
Possible CIED-LI: Symptoms/signs of systemic infection AND: echocardiography consistent with lead vegetations NO major Duke microbiological criteria present OR: symptoms/signs of systemic infection AND: major Duke criteria present NO echocardiographic evidence of lead vegetations	- Consider device removal during continued observation with repeated echography and repeated blood cultures. (For details about patient evaluation, see 8. Diagnosis) - Commence intravenous empiric antibiotic therapy targeting both Gram-positive (including MRSA) and Gram-negative bacteria. - Start targeted treatment after results from blood cultures.	Continue initial iv treatment until diagnosis is established or ruled out.
CIED-associated endocarditis, CIED-IE Duke criteria for definite endocarditis satisfied, with echocardiographic evidence of valve involvement	- Device removal recommended - Commence intravenous empiric antibiotic therapy (**Table 5**) targeting both Gram-positive (including MRSA) and Gram-negative bacteria. - Start targeted treatment after results from blood cultures.	Native cardiac structures involved: 4 weeks iv Extracardiac foci (e.g. skeleton): 6 weeks iv
Probable CIED infection Occult bacteremia, neither proof of CIED infection nor alternative sources of infection but resolving after CIED extraction.	- Device removal after thorough evaluation and exclusion of alternative sources of bacteremia. - Antimicrobial treatment, as CIED-LI.	Treat as CIED-LI.

**Clinical systemic signs of infection include rigors, fever, embolic phenomena, and improvement after treatment.*
***In some guidelines, device erosion is described as an entity of its own, as this always means that the system will be infected, regardless of symptoms.*
****Consider day 1 as the first day of appropriate antimicrobials unless persistently bacteremic on therapy.*

Table 1.
Adopted from Sanoe et al. [7].

is difficult, but possible and would require a structurally normal tricuspid valve that remains normal after device extraction and no findings suspicious of pocket infection. Cases with occult bacteremia and neither proof of CIED infection nor alternative sources of infection, resolving after CIED extraction, are reasonable to title probable CIED infection. It may take time and sometimes also device removal before a definite diagnosis is established. However, the proposed categories may be relevant before that, as a way to structure early management. Clinical systemic signs of infection include rigors, fever, embolic phenomena, and improvement after treatment.

4. Epidemiology

The last decades have seen a steady increase in the number of patients with CIEDs [13–15]. Originally made up mostly of pacemaker implants, the continuing increase today is largely due to rising implantation rates of ICD and CRT devices [16]. Using current evidence to determine the true incidence of CIED infection is hard, as there is no uniform or mandatory reporting, no universal definition of how to classify the disease and many differences between studies regarding the time frame for measured incidence. Reviews of the literature suggest an overall incidence of CIED infection of 0.5–2.2%, based on different follow up periods from 6 weeks to 11 years [7]. Some studies instead report incidence per 1000 device years. Three large registry studies of pacemaker and ICD patients report 1.8-3.1 per 1000 device years [17–19].

As new surgical procedures mature, implantation volumes increase, and the operating staff becomes more skilled, it is often reasonable to expect that the incidence of complications will decrease [20]. For CIED infections however, the opposite has been the case. Despite the variations in reported incidence and technique of reporting incidence, there are consistent results from several long-term registry studies showing increasing infection rates over time [9, 13, 18, 20–22]. These studies display not only the well-known trend of increasing implantation rate, accentuated by wider indications for ICD treatment, but also an unproportional increase in CIED infections. Furthermore, they report higher incidence of infection for ICDs and CRT compared to pacemakers and for device revisions (such as upgrades or replacements) compared to *de novo* implantations [23, 24].

A clarifying example is a study of US discharge registries 1993–2008; during the 16-year study, implantation of pacemakers increased by 45% and ICDs by 504% and the total increase in all CIED implantation was 96%. The incidence of CIED infection increased by 210% to 2.41% between 1993 and 2008. The rate of infection was fairly constant up to 2004 when a marked increase occurred. The study revealed a parallel increase in four comorbidities (renal failure, heart failure, diabetes, and respiratory failure) among the patients starting in 2004 [13]. This shift also coincided fairly close in time with the introduction of new, broader indications for ICD treatment.

This resulted in speculations about comorbidities, together with the risks of more complex devices, explaining the increase in CIED infections [13]. As neither the aging population with more comorbidities nor the wider indications for ICDs are temporary phenomena, a conclusion has been that this has set the stage for further increases in CIED infection rates, making the study of risk factors more relevant than ever [14].

5. Predictors for CIED infection

Device-related infections are the result of an interaction between different types of risk factors—related to the patient, the implantation procedure, the microbe, or the device itself [11]. These factors predispose to device infection by either increasing the risk of generator or lead contamination at the time of implantation or increasing the risk of bacteremia from a distant source with hematogenous seeding of device leads [25]. Establishing risk factors is central for prevention and numerous risk factors have been identified (**Table 2**). The evidence supporting these factors varies and their combined effect is not easily quantifiable.

5.1 Risk factors related to patient, device, and procedure

A systematic review concluded that the three most consistently identified risk factors were the number of prior procedures, their complexity, and lack of antimicrobial prophylaxis [7]. The importance of antibiotic prophylaxis has also been showed in randomized controlled trials [11].

In a meta-analysis of 60 studies (180,000 patients), the most significant patient-related risk factors were diabetes mellitus, end-stage renal disease, chronic obstructive pulmonary disease, corticosteroid use, previous device infection, renal insufficiency, malignancy, and congestive heart failure. Other significant risk factors were symptomatic heart failure, preprocedural fever, anticoagulant drug use, heparin bridging, and chronic skin disorders. Procedural risk factors identified were postoperative hematoma, reintervention for lead dislodgement, device revision/replacement, lack of antibiotic prophylaxis, temporary pacing before the procedure, generator exchange, and inexperienced operator (<100 procedures). Significant

Patient-related risk factors:	Procedure-related risk factors:
Age and comorbidities	Pocket hematoma
Renal failure	Device replacement versus *de novo* implant
End stage renal disease/hemodialysis	Extended procedure
Diabetes mellitus	Inexperienced surgeon
Heart failure	Lack of prophylactic antibiotics
Chronic obstructive pulmonary disease	
Temporary pacing	**Device-related risk factors:**
Periprocedural fever (within 24 h)	History of multiple device-related procedures
Malignancy	≥2 leads
Skin disorder	ICD/CRT (compared to pacemaker)
Prior CIED infection	Epicardial lead(s)
Anticoagulation	Abandoned lead(s)
Immunosuppressive drug/stat	Recent device manipulation

Microbe-related risk factors:
S. aureus and other gram-positive cocci
Existence of central venous catheter
Postoperative wound infection

Table 2.
Risk factors for CIED infection [7, 11, 14, 25].

device-related risk factors were abdominal generator pocket, presence of epicardial leads, and positioning of two or more leads [26].

Although this meta-analysis did not show higher infection risks for ICDs compared to pacemakers, there are numerous other studies indicating such a risk, and a generally higher risk with more complex devices including CRT [18, 27–29]. Even though it is hard to exactly quantify the difference in risk of infection with an ICD or CRT compared to a pacemaker, it is clear that more complex devices should be regarded as a risk factor [11].

Several risk factors are linked to the reopening of the device pocket, for example during upgrades, which increases the risk of introducing bacteria—highlighting problems with today's frequent upgrades and recalls.

Several summaries of known risk factors attribute age as a risk factor [11, 25, 30]. However, it is not certain that it is a fully independent factor and some studies show contradicting results, for example, the meta-analysis mentioned above [17, 26]. As old age has been consistently associated to more co-morbidities and more complex devices, we have chosen to list "old age and comorbidities" as a risk factor [11]. There are also uncertainties regarding male sex that has been listed as a risk factor of infection in a few studies [7]. Reopening of the pocket is linked to several risk factors.

5.2 Microbe-related risk factors

Studies point to a risk of CIED infection as high as 35–45% when *Staphylococcus aureus* (*S. aureus*) is found in blood cultures [8, 29], 30% with other Gram-positive cocci [31], and 6% with blood cultures with Gram-negative bacteria [32]. Hence, the finding of either *S. aureus* or other Gram-positive cocci in blood cultures is in itself a substantial risk factor for CIED infection [7].

5.3 Risk factors associated with early versus late onset infections

Studies on infections of ICD systems suggest that there are differences between risk factors as to whether they increase the risk of early onset infections (within 6 months of implantation) or later infection. In one study, epicardial leads and postoperative wound complications, such as pocket hematoma, were associated with early infection while the length of hospitalization and chronic obstructive pulmonary disease was associated with later infection. A more general interpretation of this has been suggested; circumstances that increase the probability of pocket contamination in the postoperative period are more likely to be associated with early onset infection, while overall poor health of the patient increases the risk of late onset infection [33]. Attempts have also been made to find useful differences between pathogens related to early versus late onset infections, yet without clinically significant findings [34]. Although these efforts to describe patterns, typical of early versus late infections, can increase the understanding of the pathogenesis and prevention, there are yet no simple implications for management or other obvious clinical benefits of making such a division.

6. Mortality

Reviews of current evidence have found all-cause mortality to be substantial, ranging from 0% to 35%, with big variation probably due to different proportions of patient comorbidities between the studies and differences related to devices or the definition of CIED infection [7]. The high mortality figures do not only reflect the acute effects of the infection; a high proportion of the reported deaths are related to cardiac and other noninfection causes. This is also coherent with the observation that mortality is up to threefold higher when longer follow-up periods are compared to in-hospital or 30-day mortality [7]. Another observation has been

Patient-related risk factors	Procedure-related risk factors
Abnormal renal function	CRT device
Older age	Complicated device removal
Abnormal right ventricular function	De novo implant
Corticosteroid therapy	Epicardial right ventricular pacing system in those undergoing reimplantation
Endocarditis	Late removal (versus immediate)
Heart failure	System upgrade/revision
Length of time lead in-situ	
Medical therapy	
Metastatic malignancy	
Moderate/severe tricuspid regurgitation	
Pathogen other than a coagulase negative Staphylococcus	
Pre-reimplantation elevation of C-reactive protein	
Systemic embolization	
Thrombocytopenia on admission	
Adapted from Sandoe et al [7].	

Table 3.
Risk factors for mortality in CIED infections.

that studies including only CIED endocarditis report higher mortality (25–29%) than studies of infections localized to the device pocket [7].

Studies of mortality often focus on finding risk factors of mortality, and the most frequently reported appear to be abnormal renal function, endocarditis, and old age [35–37]. Conditions often associated with endocarditis (systemic embolization, tricuspid regurgitation) have also been noted as risk factors of mortality. Another risk factor is the identified microbe, where *S. aureus* is associated with an increased mortality [38, 39].

Table 3 shows risk factors for mortality in CIED infection as presented by Sandoe et al. [7]. Included are also factors related to device types and whether the device is extracted or if the patient receives medical therapy alone. This is discussed further under "Management", but in short, device removal is clearly associated to lower mortality [40]. Although there are possible fatal complications from device removal, the mortality associated with delaying this procedure is even higher [41]. Therefore, there is no indication for extraction as strong as infection [11, 42].

7. Pathogenesis

There are two basic mechanisms of infection, either bacterial contamination at the time of implant or hematogenous seeding of the device during bacteremia from a distant focus of infection [5].

Excluding rare cases of contamination during manufacturing, it can occur perioperatively by anyone handling the device or via the air of the operation theater. Without ventilation with laminar flow, it is likely that coagulase-negative staphylococci on skin squamae, either from the patient or any of the operating staff, are present in the air. An example of this is the *en passant* finding in one study where 14 unused sterile leads were placed on the operation table during a CIED implantation. One of the leads was positive for *Staphylococcus epidermidis* after culturing [7, 43]. During implantation and possible later manipulations or revisions, skin incisions always carry the risk of skin flora contaminating the wound and eventually the device [7, 20]. It is a common notion that most CIED infections are the result of contamination at the time of implantation, which is supported by the proven effect of surgical site prophylaxis [16].

The alternative, and less common, pathway involves hematogenous seeding from a distant focus. In this case, the type of pathogen is critical to the risk of infection with *S. aureus* conferring the highest risk, whereas the risk of CIED infection from gram-negative bacteremia is low [20].

The common conceptual separation of local device pocket infection from infection involving leads and bacteremia serves a purpose for describing pathogenesis or planning preventive strategies. In practice, it is however often hard to differentiate between the two [5]. Once the generator pocket is infected, bacteria can migrate along the leads to finally reach intracardiac structures. And although pocket infection most often is due to perioperative contamination, hematogenous seeding to the pocket is also a possibility [14]. The eventual consequence of CIED infection can be the forming of vegetations anywhere on the lead and on the tricuspid valve as well as the right atrial or ventricular endocardium. Septic pulmonary embolism is a frequent complication of device endocarditis [5].

However, pathogenesis cannot be reduced to blood stream or wound contamination. It is the result of specific interactions between the device, the microbe, and the host [14]. Risk factors related to the patient (host) and device have been discussed in earlier sections. Additionally, there are specific device factors related to surface features and chemical interactions between pathogens and devices affecting pathogen adherence. The development of devices with better surface properties in this regard is an important topic under current exploration, although not currently relevant in clinical practice, and therefore beyond the scope of this chapter [7, 11, 16, 20]. Finally, there are specific virulence factors, all related to microbial ability to adhere to device surfaces that are crucial for establishing CIED infection. The most important of these is the ability to form biofilm [20, 25, 44]. This reduces the effectiveness of the normal immune system response to infection, supplies a barrier against antibiotic penetration, and (by metabolic downregulation) makes bacteria less susceptible to antibiotics.

8. Diagnosis

The signs and symptoms of CIED infection depend on the location of the infected part of the device, but establishing the diagnosis can sometimes be challenging with a variety of manifestations. Fever is present in most cases. It is reasonable to always consider device infection for patients with CIEDs and unexplained fever, keeping in mind that a blunted fever response is common among the elderly [5]. In some cases, with typical symptoms of localized generator pocket infection, diagnosing CIED infection is simple. In other cases, the symptoms can be extremely vague despite extensive infection, often resulting in diagnostic delays. As with other types of endocarditis, diagnosis is not built on a single test, but rather evaluation of a pattern of signs and investigations where echocardiography and blood cultures play a fundamental role. Sometimes, *S. aureus* bacteremia can be the only sign of device infection [5]. A central recommendation in guidelines is also that the patient with suspected CIED infection should be evaluated by a multidisciplinary team [14].

8.1 Clinical presentation

The most common type of CIED infection (~60%) is a generator pocket infection with symptoms of localized inflammation including erythema, pain, swelling, warmth, erosion, and purulent drainage or skin dehiscence [45]. In less than half of these cases, there are also systemic signs of infection or positive blood cultures [25, 45]. Often, these signs are easily identified, motivating the patient to seek medical attention. But sometimes, the symptoms are more subtle, presenting soon after implantation and thereby hard to differentiate from pure postoperative inflammation, skin reactions to dressings, disinfection agents, and sutures or a restricted and superficial infection [7, 11].

A second major manifestation is that of infection affecting either cardiac valves, device leads, or a combination of these two (CIED-IE or CIED-LI). This accounts for 10–23% of all CIED infections [25, 46]. Many of these patients have typical signs of systemic infection, presenting with fever, rigors, malaise, fatigue, or anorexia. Most, but not all, show positive blood cultures [11, 45]. Parallel symptoms of device pocket infection make the diagnosis easier, but this is not always the case. Instead, the presence of a CIED is often disregarded by the first doctor seeing the patient [24]. Major diagnostic tools recommended by guidelines are cardiac imaging, repeated blood cultures and use of the modified Duke criteria (**Table 4**) [7, 12].

In the case of cardiac vegetations, the tricuspid valve is the most common site, but vegetations may also appear on both the pulmonic and left-sided valves. *S. aureus* is the most common pathogen. In this patient group, it is common with symptoms or radiographic findings indicating septic embolism to the lungs (~40%) as well as other organs (18%), and occasionally distant abscess formation [46–48]. Possible embolic phenomena are important to keep in mind, as secondary foci of infection, such as vertebral osteomyelitis or discitis, can be the main symptom presented by the patient [7, 47]. Other possible sites of metastatic abscesses are brain, liver, kidney, and spleen. In some cases, it will be hard to distinguish if a distal site of infection is the result of

Duke criteria	
Major	**Definite endocarditis**
Blood culture positive for IE	- 2 major criteria; or
Evidence of endocardial involvement	- 1 major criterion and 3 minor criteria; or
Echocardiogram positive for IE	- 5 minor criteria
New valvular regurgitation (worsening of pre-existent murmur not sufficient)	
	Possible endocarditis:
Minor	- 1 major and 1 minor criterion
Predisposition (predisposing heart condition, iv drug use)	-3 minor criteria
Fever (>38°C)	
Vascular phenomena, major arterial emboli, septic pulmonary infarcts, mycotic aneurysm, intracranial hemorrhage, conjunctival hemorrhage, and Janeway lesions	
Immunologic phenomena: glomerulonephritis, Osler's nodes, Roth´s spots, and rheumatoid factor	
Microbiological evidence: positive blood culture but does not meet a major criterion or serological evidence of active infection with organism consistent with IE	
Microorganisms consistent with IE: (positive results from 2 separate blood cultures required)	
- *Streptococcus viridans*	
- *Streptococcus bovis*	
- HACEK group (*Haemophilus* spp., *Aggregatibacter*, *Cardiobacterium*, *Eikenella*, *Kingella*)	
- *Staphylococcus aureus*	
- Community-acquired enterococci, in the absence of a primary focus	
Or:	
Microorganisms consistent with IE from persistently positive blood cultures, defined as follows: at least two positive cultures of blood samples drawn >12 h apart, or	
all of three or a majority of ≥4 separate cultures (with first and last sample drawn at least 1 h apart)	
Single positive blood culture for *Coxiella burnetii* or antiphase 1 IgG antibody titer >1:800	

Table 4.
The Duke criteria, adapted from Li et al. [12].

hematogenous seeding from a cardiac device or if the opposite is true [25]. Less than 10% present with septic shock, usually caused by virulent pathogens such as *S. aureus* or *Pseudomonas aeruginosa* [7, 44]. Less virulent pathogens are generally associated with a more subacute or chronic presentation. In rare cases, this can be coupled with immune-complex mediated conditions such as nephritis or vasculitis [44].

In contrast to the diversity of symptoms mentioned above, occult bacteremia (or in rare cases fungemia) without localized symptoms at the generator pocket represents a diagnostic challenge primarily by the absence of findings [11, 25]. Studies indicate that laboratory abnormalities are present in less than half of the cases of CIED infection, hence normal laboratory results should not rule out CIED infection [9, 25]. Distant foci of infection could result in hematogenous seeding of the device but should not always be interpreted as evidence of actual CIED infection. To avoid misdiagnosis and unnecessary and riskful extractions, an algorithm for managing bacteremia among CIED patients has been presented by DeSimone and Sohail [49].

Except for these three main presentations, there are occasional cases of device erosion through the skin with neither positive blood cultures nor any other local inflammatory changes. Usually, erosion is a slow process of fat necrosis and migration from deeper layers of the skin and seldom presents shortly after implantation.

The exact cause often remains unclear but can be low grade device infection, other local infections or mechanical factors alone [11]. Whenever a generator or lead has eroded through the skin, the whole device system should be regarded as infected [7].

8.2 Diagnostic challenges

Beyond the typical and distinct clinical manifestations, there are also many cases with scarce or misleading symptoms. One study reports that many diagnostic delays are related to the fact that CIED infection was not considered in the original differential diagnosis, for instance, when device patients present with mainly respiratory or rheumatic symptoms that are interpreted as bronchitis [5, 47]. Other reasons for delay could be that possible hints about the diagnosis were disregarded, for instance positive blood cultures for *Staphylococcus epidermidis* first considered to represent contamination. Sometimes, the diagnosis was taken into consideration, but wrongly excluded without adequate investigations, such as a negative transthoracic echocardiography (TTE) being interpreted as sufficient for excluding the diagnosis [47].

8.3 Microbiology and adequate sampling

A series of studies consistently show that staphylococci and Gram-positive bacteria in general are responsible for most CIED infections. Methicillin resistance among *S. aureus* has been reported to various extents, depending on geographic and individual factors [5]. We found the figures of the prevalence of respective pathogens fairly consistent with the results of prior studies and systematic reviews [7, 9, 11, 25, 45, 47, 50–52]. Consistent are also reports of negative cultures despite clinical infection. A reason for this may be previous antibiotic treatment and fastidious microbes [25]. Negative blood cultures should be interpreted with caution and exclusion of infection should not rely exclusively on cultures.

At least two sets of blood cultures (including aerobic and anaerobic cultures) are recommended before starting antibiotic therapy. For patients presenting with acute symptoms, ideally the two sets should be taken at different times within 1 h from peripheral sites. If the clinical presentation is chronic/subacute, guidelines recommend three sets of cultures to be taken from peripheral sites with >6 h between each sample, before antibiotic therapy is started [7]. The point of taking multiple cultures with certain waiting periods is hopes of improved sensitivity and the ability to differentiate between transient and persistent bacteremia. Consistently positive blood cultures with the same pathogen are highly indicative of CIED infection. If purulent drainage is present from the device pocket, a culture can be very useful and more sensitive than other pocket cultures. Percutaneous aspiration of the pocket should, however, not be done because of the risk of introducing microorganisms and possibly causing device infection [14]. When a device is removed, device pocket swabs and tissue culture as well as both proximal and distal lead cultures should be obtained [11]. The lead-tip cultures should be interpreted with caution if extracted through an infected device pocket because of the risk of contamination. Possible femoral extraction would reduce this risk. The clinical situation when lead tip cultures interpreted as unequivocally significant is when there is no sign of pocket infection [25, 50]. After device removal, the recommendation is to obtain new blood cultures after 48–72 h.

8.4 Cardiac imaging

Echocardiography is a cornerstone for diagnosing CIED infection, visualizing lead or endocardial vegetations, and estimating valve regurgitation and vegetation size. TTE is superior for pericardial effusion and estimations of ventricular function and pulmonary pressure. TTE is also convenient for repeated monitoring of vegetations and cardiac function before or after extraction. Transesophageal echocardiography (TEE) is however superior for diagnosing lead and endocardial infection (CIED-LI, CIED-IE), visualizing vegetations, valves and parts of the lead that are difficult to see by TTE. It is also superior for visualizing left-sided endocarditis and perivalvular abscesses. For the diagnosis of CIED-IE, the sensitivity of TEE is >90%, compared to 22–43% for TTE [7]. Hence, both modalities should be used, but in this complimentary manner. Despite the high sensitivity of TEE, it is important keeping in mind that a normal echocardiography does not completely rule out the possibility of CIED infection [5, 7, 10, 11, 14, 30].

It has been demonstrated that TEE cannot distinguish vegetations from sterile thrombi [14, 30]. In studies validating TEE, 5–10% of identified lead masses, first described as vegetations, were concluded to represent incidentally found thrombi [53, 54]. This underlines the importance of a thorough multidisciplinary evaluation using the sum of all findings to assess the patient; masses found on leads in patients without symptoms of infection or positive blood cultures should consequently not be treated with device extraction and antibiotics, but possibly anticoagulants [10].

New imaging modalities (^{18}F-FDG positron emission tomography/computerized tomography, ^{99m}TcHMPAO-WBC) have been studied in a few early reports suggesting slightly increased sensitivity compared to TEE and possibly a high negative predictive value. Limited evidence of their possible added clinical value, high costs, and limited availability so far has not resulted in recommended routine use and guidelines describe them as a possibility to consider in selected and complicated cases. The same approach is recommended for intracardiac echocardiography that possibly may enhance diagnostic accuracy, but just like TEE, is unable to distinguish thrombi from infective vegetations [7, 11, 30].

The role of ordinary chest X-ray has not been studied specifically. Guidelines recommend chest X-ray for patients presenting with acute symptoms as a baseline image during circumstances when full medical records may not be available [7]. Chest computerized tomography or pulmonary angiography can contribute in complicated diagnostic processes by finding septic emboli that constitute a minor Duke criterion.

9. Management

Successful management of CIED infection is dependent on complete and prompt device removal, long antimicrobial treatment, and reimplantation if the device is still indicated. In a few cases, device removal may not be possible, which substantially reduces the probability of curing the infection. There is a lack of randomized controlled trials to guide management of CIED infection. Most of today's practice is based on the results of observational studies or clinical expertise [25, 55].

In the case of suspected CIED infection, initially two or three blood cultures (depending on urgency) should be taken, followed by the initiation of empiric antibiotic treatment. After that, it is important to determine whether the device should be removed or not [7].

9.1 Device removal

Results from several retrospective studies have shown that complete and early device removal (despite its rare but potentially fatal complications) together with antibiotics is more effective than medical therapy alone with dramatically lower figures for mortality and infection relapse [9, 41, 56]. A multivariate analysis of a large CIED infection cohort showed a sevenfold increase in 30-day mortality for patients treated with medical therapy alone compared to the combination with device removal [41]. In a large retrospective study of patients in Cleveland, 97% (pocket infection and CIED-IE) were cured by extraction combined with antibiotics [45]. Therefore, complete device removal is the general recommendation for established CIED infection [7, 11].

What is the implication of this for our previous presented clinical categories? The most benign case is that of post-implantation inflammation, where the device should not be removed. However, a close follow-up is important: what is first perceived as inflammation can later be interpreted as early symptoms of infection [7]. If symptoms instead are accordant with device pocket infection (complicated or uncomplicated), device removal is inevitable. That is also the case for the more extensive infections, definite CIED-LI and CIED-IE.

Remaining are two diagnostically more difficult categories: "possible CIED-LI" and "probable CIED infection" (occult bacteremia) for which guidelines recommend that device removal is considered while the patient is under continued observation with repeated echocardiography and blood cultures. Evaluation by physicians with specific expertise in CIED infection is always recommended when a diagnosis is established, but is also an option for *suspected* infection if the investigation is complicated [11]. Additional radiology could strengthen a diagnosis in the case of complications of CIED infection such as septic arthritis, spine infection, pulmonary embolism, vein thrombosis, or metastatic abscess [7, 25]. If available, new modalities such as FDG-positron emission tomography/computerized tomography might play a role by adding information in complex cases. In the case of bacteremia of an unknown source, all removable non-CIED sources of infection (such as intravenous lines) should be taken out [11]. A single positive blood culture without other symptoms is not sufficient for immediate device removal but the identified pathogen can give vital information. As mentioned in previous sections, CIED infection is more likely with Gram-positive bacteremia. *S. aureus* should not be neglected and instead always regarded as a possible pathogen, requiring further investigations in search of a source [11]. In the case of *S. aureus* bacteremia where there are no clinical or echocardiographic findings supporting CIED infection, earlier American Heart Association guidelines have mentioned six parameters associated with CIED infection [14]:

- Relapsing bacteremia after finished antibiotic course.
- No other source of bacteremia is identified.
- Bacteremia persisting >24 h.
- The CIED is an ICD.
- The patient has a prosthetic valve.
- Bacteremia occurs within three months of device implantation.

A scientific statement from the Heart Rhythm Society stresses that early diagnosis and lead extraction Within three days of diagnosis were associated with lower mortality in a small study [11, 40]. British guidelines recommend extraction as early as possible, but not later than within two weeks of diagnosis [7]. CIED infection can also occur for surgically implanted devices with epicardial leads. Basically, what has been stated for ordinary leads is also valid for epicardial leads. Complete device removal is recommended, after analyzing the risk of surgery for the individual patient compared to the risk from CIED infection. For localized pocket infection though, a practice of cutting the epicardial leads, only extracting the portion close to the pocket is used [11].

9.2 Antibiotic treatment

For patients with suspected post-operative inflammation, the use of antibiotics is controversial. It is reasonable to first consider if continued observation is sufficient. If needed, guidelines recommend a short oral course [7]. For all other clinical categories, some antimicrobial treatment is recommended. A multidisciplinary approach involving infectious disease specialists and individual adaptations depending on the patient's risk factors and comorbidities is essential.

A basic principle is to start with broad empirical treatment, if systemic infection is suspected. At this stage, treatment should target both Gram-positive, including methicillin-resistant *S. aureus* (MRSA), and Gram-negative bacteria [11]. The duration of antibiotic treatment is counted from the first negative culture after device removal and depends on a number of factors including the specific pathogen, extent of device infection, and existence of complications, if the device has been successfully removed or not. As with other parts of management, there is a lack of solid evidence and the choice of antibiotics and treatment durations are primarily based on expert opinion and experience [11]. Examples of regimens from current guidelines are provided in **Tables 1** and **5**, but it is also important to always consider local resistance patterns. The category "uncomplicated device pocket infection" by definition does not include systemic infection. However, some of these patients will eventually develop sepsis and therefore it is reasonable to start empiric therapy. Once a pathogen is identified through cultures, treatment should be modified accordingly.

9.3 Reimplantation

After removal of infected devices, it is crucial to always thoroughly reassess the need for a new CIED. Some patients no longer meet an original indication because of improvements in heart rhythm or function. Others have a strong personal opinion and do not accept a new implantation [11]. For some patients, another type of device can reduce possible risks of infection relapse (device downgrade and alternative devices are further described under prevention). The percentage of patients with CIED infection not requiring a replacement device has ranged from 13 to 52% in different studies [25].

Diagnosis/scenario	**Suggested antibiotics**	**Dose***	
Pocket infection, uncomplicated	Vancomycin or daptomycin or teicoplanin	1 g q12h iv 4 mg/kg q24h iv 6 mg/kg to a maximum of 1 g given at 0.12 an 24 h and then q24h	
CIED-LI, CIED-IE, or complicated pocket infection, pending blood cultures, e.g. in sepsis	Vancomycin AND meropenem or daptomycin AND meropenem	1 g q12 iv 1 g q8h 8–10 mg/kg q24h 1 g q8h iv	(appropriate spectrum, but risk of nephrotoxicity) (gentamicin in high dose, according to local guidelines, may be appropriate depending on local epidemiology) (less risk of nephrotoxicity than vancomycin)
CIED-LI or CIED-IE or complicated pocket infection with negative blood cultures	Vancomycin AND gentamicin or daptomycin AND gentamicin	1 g q12h iv 1 mg/kg q12h iv 8–10 mg/kg q24h 1 mg/kg q12h iv	(appropriate spectrum but risk of nephrotoxicity)

*iv: intravenously, q8h: every 8 hours, q12h: every 12 hours, and q24h: every 24 hours.**All doses may require adjustment due to impaired renal function.*

Table 5.
Examples of guideline regimens for empiric antibiotic treatment.

Clearance of infection is a prerequisite before hardware can be reimplanted. The optimal timing of reimplantation is however not known as no prospective trials have been done. According to recommendations from the Heart Rhythm Society, it is reasonable to await a 72 h period of negative blood cultures before reimplantation, also mentioning that there are single center studies indicating that reimplantation the same day as device extraction is possible for isolated pocket infections [11]. The existence of undrained abscesses or other sources of infection would demand further postponing of these suggested waiting times. It is also recommended that a new device is placed on the contralateral side, an attempt to reduce the risk of seeding the new device from a prior tissue infection [9]. If remains of valvular infection are suspected, the waiting period should be extended to at least 14 days according to the European Society of Cardiology guidelines [5]. British guidelines, illustrating that there is no unanimity here, recommends reimplantation to whenever possible be delayed until signs of infection have resolved suggesting 7–10 days [7].

The pacemaker-dependent patient poses a special challenge. Some form of temporary pacing is needed as a bridge to reimplantation. Common problems of traditional temporary pacing are frequent loss of capture, undersensing, and that the systems in general are large and inconvenient, all this confining the patent to stay immobilized in a hospital bed during antibiotic treatment before reimplantation. Studies of "semi-permanent" systems with active fixation leads and an external reusable pacemaker have shown that this practice is safe, reduces hospital stays, and makes the patient more mobile [11, 57]. However, these studies have so far only included a smaller number of patients and therefore are not able to rule out that the risks for relapsing infection earlier observed with temporary pacing still holds [58]. Therefore, all sorts of temporary pacing should still be regarded as a risk factor and avoided if possible, even though this semi-permanent technique probably is a way to reduce adverse events [5]. For ICD-patients with high risk of sudden cardiac death, the wearable cardioverter defibrillator can be a promising option. This noninvasive device is worn under normal clothing safely and effectively treats ventricular tachyarrhythmias, thus offering bridging to ICD reimplantation, (if the indication still holds) without increasing the risk of CIED infection relapse [59].

9.4 Management when device removal is not possible

Despite all known benefits of device removal, there are a small proportion of the patients that either decline device removal or are considered medically unfit for device removal. For many of these patients, it is likely that extraction will require surgical intervention and often they may be more or less dependent on a device (for instance CRT) that is not considered possible to reimplant. They may also have other, permanent, sources of infection or a short life expectancy [11]. There is not much evidence to guide the management of these patients, but various smaller reports have described very varied outcomes. Some describe patients being cured with medical therapy alone. Others describe the strategy of partial device removal (only generator), which is possible for nonpacemaker-dependent patients, with cure rates in a wide range from 13 to 71%. There are also reports of ICD patients with 100% failure [7].

British guidelines include regimens for attempts to salvage devices with medical therapy alone [7]. These consist of different combinations of antibiotics (for instance daptomycin and vancomycin), aiming to break through biofilm and are based on combinations that have salvaged infected non-CIED prosthetic materials and other devices. The duration of therapy is often 6 weeks. There is no known test to evaluate this therapy besides observation and blood cultures after the end of a course. Infection relapse is equivalent to a failure to salvage the device. In that case (unless the decision about device removal does not change), the only option is a palliative strategy of life-long suppressive antibiotic treatment. Patients in this group are usually cardiovascularly stable and have responded well to antibiotics with clinical improvement and cleared bloodstream infection. This strategy can obviously only be applied to a few selected patients and the outcome is also unclear. Compared to curative strategies, this should be regarded as a last resort [11].

9.5 Risks associated with device removal

Device removal should be performed in specialized centers with expertise in the procedure and acute cardiac surgery backup available [30]. Percutaneous procedures have become the most used method as procedural risks are lower compared to open surgery. In case of failures with a percutaneous technique, a conversion to open surgery is common. Removal of leads engrafted in cardiac tissue can be dangerous. Over time, fibrous anchoring tends to develop between leads and vascular and cardiac structures. Inter-lead anchoring is also common. The major procedural complications are related to these anchorings and accidental tears or perforations of either the superior vena cava or parts of the myocardial wall with resulting dramatic bleeding and tamponade. Lead fracture often requires shifts to open surgery and can cause life threatening arrhythmias. To reduce risks, new techniques with locking stylets, photoablation of fibrous attachments, and less invasive methods aided by thoracoscopy have been developed [30, 60, 61]. In experienced centers, procedure mortality is low, between 0.1 and 0.6% [5]. If removal employs this type of special equipment, or concerns a lead implanted more than a year ago, the procedure is referred to as *extraction* as compared to *explantation* [11].

A number of procedural risk factors have been identified one of the more evident being elapsed time since lead implantation, which is related to the fibrous anchorings. Other risk factors are female sex, multiple leads (lead-lead anchoring), operator inexperience, and radiological findings of calcification involving leads. ICD is a risk factor as the device is bigger and more complex. In particular, the coils are suspected of stimulating fibrotic growth between device and myocardium and some extracting operators choose to only implant single coils for this reason [60].

In the case of very large vegetations, there is risk of pulmonary embolism. For very large vegetation, a shift to open surgery is common. There is uncertainty about how large vegetations should be for this shift to benefit the patient. Guidelines state that additional data are needed and recommend individualized decisions for vegetations >2 cm in diameter [5].

10. Prevention

As CIED infection results in substantial morbidity and mortality as well as high and rising costs for health care systems, good prevention is essential. The first subsection here is valid for all device patients. The following, covering secondary prevention, is specific for CIED infection patients. Being an essential and integrated part of all CIED infection management, it is not always specifically referred to as prevention. Finally, we give an outline of new therapies and devices with possible implications for all potential devices.

10.1 Primary prevention

Before implantation, the patient must be evaluated for clinical signs of infection. Fever during the last 24 h before implantation is a risk marker for later CIED infection. Signs of systemic infection should always result in elective implantations being postponed and acute procedures should be avoided until the infectious episode is resolved [7]. Perioperative antibiotics reduce the risk of infection. A randomized controlled study was interrupted after having enrolled 649 patients, showing an infection rate of 3.4% for the placebo group versus 0.6% in the antibiotics group [11]. When risk markers are studied, neglected perioperative antibiotics are one of the more consistent predictors of infection risk. Intravenous administration of a cephalosporin or penicillinase resistant penicillin 1 h before procedural start or vancomycin 2 h before start are commonly used [11]. Repeated dosing after skin closure or general postoperative antibiotic use is not recommended. Except for TYRX™ (see Section 10.3), there is so far no support in evidence for local installation of antibiotics or antiseptics into the device pocket [7, 62].

Implantation should ideally take place in a designated CIED laboratory fulfilling requirements for ventilation suitable for device surgery. This is underlined by the fact that it is not unusual with perioperative CIED contamination today and many CIEDs are implanted in catheterization laboratories with lower ventilation requirements than operation theaters [7]. Implantation should be carried out with an aseptic technique, in an environment observing operating theater discipline. Alcoholic chlorhexidine (2%) should be used to prepare the skin over the operative site. Devices and surgical equipment should be left uncovered for the minimum possible time [7].

Risk of infection is also related to operator experience and the aggregated operation volumes of different centers—at least it has been shown that very small volumes are related to higher risk of complications: a study of Medicare recipients showed that physicians implanting 1–10 ICDs annually had higher complication rates than physicians implanting more than 29 devices [63]. A US registry study found a complication rate of 3.8% at centers performing fewer than 24 implants a year compared to 3.1% at centers implanting more than 110 devices a year [64]. British guidelines stress the importance of supervision of junior operators (with lower operation volumes) by senior operators. They also speculate about if a lack of supervision is more common for generator exchange procedures, which have a higher risk of infection than de novo implants, but often are viewed as simple and "straightforward procedures" [7].

Postoperative hematomas are a consistently found risk factor. If possible, antithrombotic treatment and anticoagulation should be discontinued prior to the procedure. If a pause in anticoagulation is not deemed possible, it is however better to continue with ordinary warfarin doses than discontinuing and trying to bridge with heparin as this is related to a significant increase in pocket hematomas [7]. As for new oral anticoagulants (NOACs), there are less data, but studies suggest that there is no difference in pocket hematoma between interrupted and continued NOAC regimens [65].

10.2 Secondary prevention

The most effective preventive measure against CIED infection is to avoid unnecessary CIED implants in the first place. For patients with CIED infection, a reassessment of the risks and benefits of the device before reimplantation is crucial, and a significant proportion of the patients do actually not meet indications for reimplantation. As the risk is also associated with various properties of the device, this reevaluation can also result in a device downgrade, for instance from a more complex to a simpler device, or from two defibrillator coils to one on an ICD. An option is also to change from transvenous leads to epicardial leads, or more commonly, to choose some of the newer devices described below.

A general principle of CIED infections is to remove all hardware, but if this is not possible, as much as possible should be removed. Examples of the latter is the isolated removal of the generator for nonpacemaker-dependent patients who refuse lead extraction or the practice of cutting the leads and removing the proximal part together with the generator when epicardial lead extraction is regarded too risky, all based on the presumption that the generator accounts for the biggest infection burden in a CIED and that its removal is a simple procedure compared to lead extraction.

The risk of infection is less with peripheral cannulae than cuffed central venous catheters and patients can be treated with peripheral cannulae for very long periods, as long as the cannulae are changed every 72 h [66]. In fact, the risk of infection for any vascular access increases with time in situ. A central venous catheter also increases the risk of venous thrombosis reducing access options for future CIED placement. For some patients, though, siting cannulae can become very complicated and alternative strategies are needed as oral administration during CIED infection is not a safe procedure. Peripherally installed catheters (PICC or "midline") may in that case be a better alternative than central venous catheters [7].

As mentioned in previous sections, temporary pacing with an intravenous pacing wire is associated with higher risk of infection relapse and should if possible be avoided for CIED infection patients. If central venous catheters are used, potential future access sites for CIEDs (contralateral prepectoral to existing CIED) should be avoided if possible. Semi-permanent pacing with screw-in leads is probably better than traditional temporary pacing, but both techniques should be avoided unless the patient is dependent on pacing. It seems that this is not only valid for CIED infection patients (and thereby also an example of primary prevention); for acute patients, it is becoming more common to directly implant a pacemaker, rather than using temporary pacing with higher risk of future CIED infection [7, 58, 67].

10.3 Alternative device systems

A leadless pacemaker suitable for VVI-pacing can be implanted in the right ventricle through femoral venous access. It is a means of avoiding the traditional complications associated with leads or generator pockets, and studies have shown promising results with lower complication rates compared to transvenous CIEDs [68, 69]. However, to our knowledge, no randomized controlled studies have yet compared leadless and transvenous pacemakers. Also, no long-term studies have yet been completed. In situations with limited venous access as well as reimplantation after CIED infection for high risk patients, leadless pacing should be considered.

A subcutaneous ICD is an alternative to transvenous systems that can be considered as an option for reimplantation in patients with high risk of CIED infection relapse. With this system, complications related to leads or vascular access are avoided. It has proved to be as effective as an ordinary ICD in treating life-threatening arrhythmias, but it is unsuitable for patients needing pacing, resynchronization therapy, or antitachycardia pacing [70–72].

Since 2001, the noninvasive wearable cardioverter defibrillator has been available to provide temporary protection against sudden cardiac death. It safely and effectively detects and terminates ventricular arrhythmias and should be considered as a bridging therapy to ICD reimplantation. As a reassessment of the indications should take place before every reimplantation, the wearable cardioverter defibrillator also has the potential of bridging to a device downgrade [59, 73, 74].

In addition to perioperative systemic antibiotics, an antibiotic envelope (TYRX™) has been developed, wrapping the device and slowly releasing antibiotics (minocycline and rifampin) in the device pocket. A meta-analysis of five prior studies including 4490 patients showed that use of the envelope is associated with significantly lowering the CIED infection rate, although the included studies were not randomized controlled trials [75]. Other studies have particularly showed benefits among patients categorized as high risk individuals for early CIED infection (risk factors, **Table 2**) [76]. As the envelope is costly and its use is not yet routine, this selected patient group is probably the most promising to start with, although there are cost-benefit studies indicating a role for this envelope as a standard of care for all patients, at least in the context of the US health care system [77].

Current evidence does not support the use of prophylactic antibiotics for dental procedures or other invasive procedures that do not involve direct device manipulation [11].

11. Conclusions

CIED infection is a rare but severe complication. As more complex devices are implanted in patients with more co-morbidities, the infection rate is on the rise. CIED infection should always be considered in device patients with unexplained fever—the presence of *S. aureus* bacteremia is equivalent to a risk of device infection of almost 50%. Once infection is established, renal impairment, old age, and endocarditis are some of the most consistently found predictors of mortality. Although not without lethal risks, device removal is the recommended treatment in all but a few cases and should be performed in designated centers. Combined with antibiotic treatment, this can enable cure rates as high as 97% according to some studies. Reassessment of the original indication should always precede device reimplantation. Intravenous lines and temporary pacing should be avoided if possible and technical alternatives such as leadless pacemakers, subcutaneous defibrillators, and antibiotic device envelopes should be considered as means of reducing risk of reinfection.

Abbreviations

CRT	cardiac resynchronization therapy
CIED	cardiac implantable electronic devices
CIED-IE	CIED-associated infective endocarditis
CIED-LI	lead infection
ICD	implantable cardioverter defibrillator
IE	infective endocarditis
NOAC	new oral anticoagulant
MRSA	methicillin-resistant *S. aureus*
TEE	transesophageal echocardiography
TTE	transthoracic echocardiography

Author details

Måns Almqvist[1], Gustav Mattsson[1*], Robin Razmi[1] and Peter Magnusson[1,2]

1 Centre for Research and Development, Uppsala University, Sweden

2 Cardiology Research Unit, Department of Medicine, Karolinska Institutet, Stockholm, Sweden

*Address all correspondence to: gustav.mattsson@regiongavleborg.se

References

[1] Cabell CH, Jollis JG, Peterson GE, et al. Changing patient characteristics and the effect on mortality in endocarditis. Archives of Internal Medicine. 2002;**162**(1):90-94

[2] Thuny F, Grisoli D, Collart F. Management of infective endocarditis: Challenges and perspectives. Lancet. 2012;**379**:965-975

[3] Osler W. The gulstonian lectures, on malignant endocarditis. British Medical Journal. 1885;**1**(1264):577-579

[4] Statista. Global number of pacemakers in 2016 and a forecast for 2023. Available from: www.statista.com/statistics/800794/pacemakers-market-volume-in-units-worldwide/. Published 2017. [Accessed: April 4, 2019]

[5] Habib G, Lancellotti P, Antunes MJ, et al. 2015 ESC guidelines for the management of infective endocarditis. European Heart Journal. 2015;**36**:3075-3123

[6] Rundström H, Kennergren C, Andersson R, et al. Pacemaker endocarditis during 18 years in Göteborg. Scandinavian Journal of Infectious Diseases. 2004;**36**(9):674-679

[7] Sandoe JAT, Barlow G, Chambers JB, et al. Guidelines for the diagnosis, prevention and management of implantable cardiac electronic device infection. Report of a joint working party project on behalf of the British Society for Antimicrobial Chemotherapy (BSAC, host organization), British Heart Rh. The Journal of Antimicrobial Chemotherapy. 2015;**70**(2):325-359

[8] Chamis AL, PG E, Cabell CH, Greenfield RA, et al. *Staphylococcus aureus* bacteremia in patients with permanent pacemakers or implantable cardioverter-defibrillators. Circulation. 2001;**104**(9):1029-1033

[9] Sohail MR, Uslan DZ, Khan AH, et al. Management and outcome of permanent pacemaker and implantable cardioverter-defibrillator infections. Journal of the American College of Cardiology. 2007;**49**(18):1851-1859

[10] Mattucci I, Durante-Mangoni E, Tripodi M-F, et al. Current trends in the management of cardiac implantable electronic device (CIED) infections. Internal and Emergency Medicine. 2012;**8**(6):465-476

[11] Kusumoto FM, Schoenfeld MH, Wilkoff BL, et al. 2017 HRS expert consensus statement on cardiovascular implantable electronic device lead management and extraction. Heart Rhythm. 2017;**14**(12):503-551

[12] Li JS, Sexton DJ, Mick N, et al. Proposed modifications to the Duke criteria for the diagnosis of infective endocarditis. Clinical Infectious Diseases. 2000;**30**(4):633-638

[13] Greenspon AJ, Patel JD, Lau E, et al. 16-Year trends in the infection burden for pacemakers and implantable cardioverter-defibrillators in the United States: 1993-2008. Journal of the American College of Cardiology. 2011;**58**(10):1001-1006

[14] Baddour LM, Epstein AE, Erickson CC, et al. Update on cardiovascular implantable electronic device infections and their management: A scientific statement from the American Heart Association. Circulation. 2010;**121**(3):458-477

[15] Baddour LM, Cha Y, Wilson WR. Infections of cardiovascular implantable electronic devices. The New England Journal of Medicine. 2012;**367**(1):842-849

[16] Baddour LM, Freeman WK, Suri RM, et al. Cardiovascular infections. In: Braunwald's Heart Disease: A Textbook

of Cardiovascular Medicine, Vol. 2. 2015. pp. 1543-1550

[17] Johansen JB, Jørgensen OD, Møller M, et al. Infection after pacemaker implantation: Infection rates and risk factors associated with infection in a population-based cohort study of 46299 consecutive patients. European Heart Journal. 2011;**32**(8):991-998

[18] Uslan DZ, Sohail MR, St Sauver JL, et al. Permanent pacemaker and implantable cardioverter defibrillator infection: A population-based study. Archives of Internal Medicine. 2007;**167**(7):679-675

[19] Gold MR, Peters RW, Johnson JW, et al. Complications associated with pectoral cardioverter-defibrillator implantation: Comparison of subcutaneous and submuscular approaches. Journal of the American College of Cardiology. 1996;**28**(5):1278-1282

[20] Nagpal A, Baddour LM, Sohail MR. Microbiology and pathogenesis of cardiovascular implantable electronic device infections. Circulation. Arrhythmia and Electrophysiology. 2012;**5**(2):433-441

[21] Voigt A, Shalaby A, Saba S. Rising rates of cardiac rhythm management device infections in the United States: 1996 through 2003. Journal of the American College of Cardiology. 2006;**48**(3):590-591

[22] Cabell CH, Heidenreich PA, Chu VH, et al. Increasing rates of cardiac device infections among Medicare beneficiaries: 1990-1999. American Heart Journal. 2004;**147**(4):582-586

[23] Poole JE, Gleva MJ, Mela T, et al. Complication rates associated with pacemaker or implantable cardioverter-defibrillator generator replacements and upgrade procedures: Results from the REPLACE registry. Circulation. 2010;**122**(16):1553-1561

[24] Harrison JL, Prendergast BD, Sandoe JAT. Guidelines for the diagnosis, management and prevention of implantable cardiac electronic device infection. Heart. 2015;**101**(4):250-252

[25] Sohail MR, Wilson WR, Baddour LM. Infections of nonvalvular cardiovascular devices. In: Mandell, Douglas, and Bennett's Principles and Practice of Infectious Diseases. Elsevier Inc; 2014. pp. 1041-1556

[26] Polyzos KA, Konstantelias AA, Falagas ME. Risk factors for cardiac implantable electronic device infection: A systematic review and meta-analysis. Europace. 2015;**17**:767-777

[27] Nery PB, Fernandes R, Nair GM, et al. Device-related infection among patients with pacemakers and implantable defibrillators: Incidence, risk factors, and consequences. Journal of Cardiovascular Electrophysiology. 2010;**21**(7):786-790

[28] Romeyer-Bouchard C, Da Costa A, Dauphinot V, et al. Prevalence and risk factors related to infections of cardiac resynchronization therapy devices. European Heart Journal. 2010;**31**(2):203-210

[29] Uslan DZ, Dowsley TF, Sohail MR, et al. Cardiovascular implantable electronic device infection in patients with *Staphylococcus aureus* bacteremia. Pacing and Clinical Electrophysiology. 2010;**33**(4):407-413

[30] DeSimone DC, Sohail MR, Mulpuru SK. Contemporary management of cardiac implantable electronic device infection. Heart. 2019;**0**:1-5

[31] Madhavan M, Sohail MR, Friedman PA, et al. Outcomes in patients with cardiovascular implantable electronic devices and bacteremia caused by gram-positive cocci other than *Staphylococcus aureus*. Circulation. Arrhythmia and Electrophysiology. 2010;**3**(6):639-645

[32] Uslan DZ, Sohail MR, Wilson WR, et al. Frequency of permanent pacemaker or implantable cardioverter-defibrillator infection in patients with gram-negative bacteremia. Clinical Infectious Diseases. 2006;**43**(6):731-736

[33] Sohail MR, Hussain S, Le KY, et al. Risk factors associated with early-versus late-onset implantable cardioverter-defibrillator infections. Journal of Interventional Cardiac Electrophysiology. 2011;**31**(2):171-183

[34] Tayebjee MH, Joy ER, Sandoe JA. Can implantable cardiac electronic device infections be defined as "early" or "late" based on the cause of infection. Journal of Medical Microbiology. 2013;**62**(PART8):1215-1219

[35] Deharo J-C, Quatre A, Mancini J, et al. Long-term outcomes following infection of cardiac implantable electronic devices: A prospective matched cohort study. Heart. 2012;**98**(9):724-731

[36] Baman TS, Gupta SK, Valle JA, et al. Risk factors for mortality in patients with cardiac device-related infection. Circulation. Arrhythmia and Electrophysiology. 2009;**2**(2):129-134

[37] Habib A, Le KY, Baddour LM, et al. Predictors of mortality in patients with cardiovascular implantable electronic device infections. The American Journal of Cardiology. 2013;**111**(6):874-879

[38] Viola GM, Awan LL, Darouiche RO. Nonstaphylococcal infections of cardiac implantable electronic devices. Circulation. 2010;**121**(19):2085-2091

[39] Le KY, Sohail MR, Friedman PA, et al. Clinical features and outcomes of cardiovascular implantable electronic device infections due to *Staphylococcal* species. The American Journal of Cardiology. 2012;**110**(8):1143-1149

[40] Viganego F, O'Donoghue S, Eldadah Z, et al. Effect of early diagnosis and treatment with percutaneous lead extraction on survival in patients with cardiac device infections. The American Journal of Cardiology. 2012;**109**(10):1466-1471

[41] Le KY, Sohail MR, Friedman PA, et al. Impact of timing of device removal on mortality in patients with cardiovascular implantable electronic device infections. Heart Rhythm. 2011;**8**(11):1678-1685

[42] Gaynor SL, Zierer A, Lawton JS, et al. Laser assistance for extraction of chronically implanted endocardial leads: Infectious versus noninfectious indications. Pacing and Clinical Electrophysiology. 2006;**29**(12):1352-1358

[43] Klug D, Wallet F, Lacroix D, et al. Local symptoms at the site of pacemaker implantation indicate latent systemic infection. Heart. 2004;**90**(8):882-886

[44] Baddour LM, Bettmann MA, Bolger AF, et al. Nonvalvular cardiovascular device-related infections. Circulation. 2003;**108**(16):2015-2031

[45] Schmitt S, Cantillon DJ, Tarakji KG, et al. Cardiac implantable electronic device infections: Presentation, management, and patient outcomes. Heart Rhythm. 2010;**7**(8):1043-1047

[46] Sohail MR, Uslan DZ, Khan AH, et al. Infective endocarditis complicating permanent pacemaker and implantable cardioverter-defibrillator infection. Mayo Clinic Proceedings. 2008;**83**(1):46-53

[47] Klug D, Lacroix D, Savoye C, et al. Systemic infection related to endocarditis on pacemaker leads: Clinical presentation and management. Circulation. 1997;**95**(8):2098-2107

[48] Cacoub P, Leprince P, Nataf P, et al. Pacemaker infective endocarditis. The American Journal of Cardiology. 1998;**82**(4):480-484

[49] DeSimone DC, Sohail MR. Management of bacteremia in patients living with cardiovascular implantable electronic devices. Heart Rhythm. 2016;**13**(11):2247-2252

[50] Greenspon AJ, Prutkin JM, Sohail MR, et al. Timing of the most recent device procedure influences the clinical outcome of lead-associated endocarditis: Results of the MEDIC (multicenter electrophysiologic device infection cohort). Journal of the American College of Cardiology. 2012;**59**(7):681-687

[51] Grammes JA, Schulze CM, Al-Bataineh M, et al. Percutaneous pacemaker and implantable cardioverter-defibrillator lead extraction in 100 patients with intracardiac vegetations defined by transesophageal echocardiogram. Journal of the American College of Cardiology. 2010;**55**(9):886-894

[52] Kuhn C, Haverich A, Knigina L, et al. Treatment of patients with recurrent or persistent infection of cardiac implantable electronic devices. Europace. 2010;**12**(9):1275-1281

[53] Lo R, D'Anca M, Cohen T. Incidence and prognosis of pacemaker lead-associated masses: A study of 1,569 transesophageal echocardiograms. The Journal of Invasive Cardiology. 2006;**18**(12):599-601

[54] Downey BC, Juselius WE, Pandian NG. Incidence and significance of pacemaker and implantable cardioverter-defibrillator lead masses discovered during transesophageal echocardiography. Pacing and Clinical Electrophysiology. 2011;**34**(6):679-683

[55] Baddour LM, Cha Y-M, Wilson WR. Clinical practice. Infections of cardiovascular implantable electronic devices. The New England Journal of Medicine. 2012;**367**(9):842-849

[56] Del Río A, Anguera I, Miró JM, et al. Surgical treatment of pacemaker and defibrillator lead endocarditis: The impact of electrode lead extraction on outcome. Chest. 2003;**124**(4):1451-1459

[57] Kawata H, Pretorius V, Phan H, et al. Utility and safety of temporary pacing using active fixation leads and externalized re-usable permanent pacemakers after lead extraction. Europace. 2013;**15**(9):1287-1291

[58] Klug D, Balde M, Pavin D, et al. Risk factors related to infections of implanted pacemakers and cardioverter-defibrillators: Results of a large prospective study. Circulation. 2007;**116**(12):1349-1355

[59] Reek S, Burri H, Roberts PR, et al. The wearable cardioverter-defibrillator: Current technology and evolving indications. Europace. 2017;**19**:335-345

[60] Field ME, Jones SO, Epstein LM. How to select patients for lead extraction. Heart Rhythm. 2007;**4**(7):978-985

[61] Wilkoff BL, Kennergren C, Love CJ, et al. Bridge to surgery: Best practice protocol derived from early clinical experience with the bridge occlusion balloon. Federated agreement from the eleventh annual lead management symposium. Heart Rhythm. 2017;**14**(10):1574-1578

[62] Krahn AD, Longtin Y, Philippon F, et al. Prevention of arrhythmia device infection trial: The PADIT trial. Journal of the American College of Cardiology. 2018;**72**(24):3098-3109

[63] Al-Khatib SM, Lucas FL, Jollis JG, et al. The relation between patients' outcomes and the volume of cardioverter-defibrillator implantation procedures performed by physicians treating medicare beneficiaries. Journal of the American College of Cardiology. 2005;**46**(8):1536-1540

[64] Freeman JV, Wang Y, Curtis JP, et al. The relation between hospital procedure volume and complications of cardioverter-defibrillator implantation from the implantable cardioverter-defibrillator registry. Journal of the American College of Cardiology. 2010;**56**(14):1133-1139

[65] Birnie DH, Healey JS, Wells GA, et al. Continued vs. interrupted direct oral anticoagulants at the time of device surgery, in patients with moderate to high risk of arterial thrombo-embolic events (BRUISE CONTROL-2). European Heart Journal. 2018;**39**(44):3973-3979

[66] Ahmed FZ, Baig WW, Munyombwe T, et al. Vascular access strategy for delivering long-term antimicrobials to patients with infective endocarditis: Device type, risk of infection and mortality. The Journal of Hospital Infection. 2013;**83**(1):46-50

[67] Sohail MR, Uslan DZ, Khan AH, et al. Risk factor analysis of permanent pacemaker infection. Clinical Infectious Diseases. 2007;**45**(2):166-173

[68] Reddy VY, Knops RE, Sperzel J, et al. Permanent leadless cardiac pacing: Results of the LEADLESS trial. Circulation. 2014;**129**(14):1466-1471

[69] Roberts PR, Clementy N, Al Samadi F, et al. A leadless pacemaker in the real-world setting: The micra transcatheter pacing system post-approval registry. Heart Rhythm. 2017;**14**(9):1375-1379

[70] Köbe J, Reinke F, Meyer C, et al. Implantation and follow-up of totally subcutaneous versus conventional implantable cardioverter-defibrillators: A multicenter case-control study. Heart Rhythm. 2013;**10**(1):29-36

[71] Burke MC, Gold MR, Knight BP, et al. Safety and efficacy of the totally subcutaneous implantable defibrillator: 2-Year results from a pooled analysis of the IDE study and EFFORTLESS registry. Journal of the American College of Cardiology. 2015;**65**(16):1605-1615

[72] Khazen C, Magnusson P, Flandorfer J, et al. The subcutaneous implantable cardioverter-defibrillator: A tertiary center experience. Cardiology Journal;**2018**

[73] Klein HU, Meltendorf U, Reek S, et al. Bridging a temporary high risk of sudden arrhythmic death. Experience with the wearable cardioverter defibrillator (WCD). Pacing and Clinical Electrophysiology. 2010;**33**(3):353-367

[74] Feldman AM, Klein H, Tchou P, et al. Use of a wearable defibrillator in terminating tachyarrhythmias in patients at high risk for sudden death: Results of WEARIT/BIROAD. Pacing and Clinical Electrophysiology. 2004;**27**(1):4-9

[75] Koerber S, Turagam M, Winterfield J, et al. Use of antibiotic envelopes to prevent cardiac implantable electronic device infections: A meta-analysis. Journal of Cardiovascular Electrophysiology. 2018;**29**(4):609-615

[76] Kolek MJ, Patel NJ, Clair WK, et al. Efficacy of a bio-absorbable antibacterial envelope to prevent cardiac implantable electronic device infections in high-risk subjects. Journal of Cardiovascular Electrophysiology. 2015;**26**(10):1111-1116

[77] Shariff N, Eby E, Adelstein E, et al. Health and economic outcomes associated with use of an antimicrobial envelope as a standard of care for cardiac implantable electronic device implantation. Journal of Cardiovascular Electrophysiology. 2015;**26**(7):783-789